The Mood Stabiliser Patient and Family Handbook

Lithium, Valproate, Lamotrigine and Carbamazepine Explained in Plain English, from the Blood Tests to the Decisions

Timothy Sawyer Duncan

Disclaimer

This book is provided for information and education only. It is not medical advice and it is not a substitute for the care of a qualified prescriber. Nothing in this book is a reason to start, stop, or change the dose of any medication without the involvement of the clinician responsible for your care. Regulatory guidance, particularly the guidance governing valproate, changes; the guidance described in this book is dated in the text and should be checked against current sources before it is relied upon.

The case studies in this book are composites. Names, ages, occupations, clinical details, and circumstances have been changed or invented. No case describes a real identifiable person, and any resemblance to an actual patient is coincidental.

The author and publisher make no representations or warranties with respect to the accuracy or completeness of the contents of this book and specifically disclaim any implied warranties of merchantability or fitness for a particular purpose. Neither the author nor the publisher shall be liable for any loss of profit or any other commercial damages, including but not limited to special, incidental, consequential, personal, or other damages. The reader assumes all risk in acting on the information contained in this book.

First Edition, 2026.

ISBN: 979-8-90599-303-9

Table of Contents

Preface

There is a folded piece of paper inside the box. You have probably read it once, in the way people read these things, standing at a kitchen counter with the kettle on. It lists side effects in descending order of frequency. It tells you what to do if you miss a dose. It has a section about pregnancy that is either two sentences or two pages depending on which drug you are holding.

It does not tell you which of the four drugs is best.

That is not an oversight. A patient information leaflet is a legal document about one product, written by the company that makes it, and it is structurally incapable of saying that a different company's product might suit you better. So the single most important question a person can ask, which is why this one and not one of the others, is the one question the paper in the box is guaranteed not to answer.

That is what this book is for.

What This Book Is About

Four drugs. Lithium, valproate, lamotrigine, and carbamazepine.

It is not a book about bipolar disorder. There are good books about bipolar disorder and this is not one of them. You will not find much here about what causes it, what it feels like, how to explain it to your employer, or what therapy helps. Those are real subjects and they are somebody else's.

This is a book about what is in your hand. What it does, what it does not do, what it costs you, what the blood tests are actually looking for, what the rules around it mean, and where the evidence for all of that is strong, weak, or contested. Where the field genuinely disagrees, this book says so rather than picking the reassuring side. There are places in here where the honest answer is that nobody knows, and I have written those out rather than smoothing them over, because a reader who is told a confident answer to an unsettled question has been given something worse than nothing.

Who It Is For

Three people, and the book keeps all three in view.

If you take one of these drugs, this is written for you first. It assumes you are an intelligent adult who has been handed a leaflet and a six-monthly appointment and left to work out the rest.

If you love someone who does, Chapter 13.0 is addressed directly to you and the rest of the book is worth your time as well. You have better data than the clinic does about several of the things in here, and nobody has ever told you that.

If you work in mental health, particularly as a nurse or a peer supporter, the parts of this that will be most useful to you are the ones about the gaps: the sampling times nobody records, the calcium nobody checks, the sertraline nobody has reviewed in nine years. Those are not failures of knowledge. They are failures of process, and they are visible from where you stand.

How to Use It

The chapters run in an order and the order means something. The first five are the drugs themselves. The middle four are the things that go wrong from outside. Chapters 9.0 through 12.0 are the four long arguments: kidneys, thyroid, weight, pregnancy. The last three are about living with this rather than starting it.

You do not have to read it in order and most people will not. If you have just been handed a prescription, start with the chapter for your drug and then read Chapter 2.0. If you have been on lithium for fifteen years, start at Chapter 9.0. If you are the person watching, start at 13.0.

The appendices are the working end of the book. They are meant to be photocopied, torn out, written on, and taken to appointments. Appendix B in particular exists because of a fact established in Chapter 2.0, which is that the trend across a decade is the clinically interesting object and no single clinician in your care will ever have seen the whole of it.

The One Rule

Nothing in this book is a reason to change a dose without a prescriber.

That sentence is going to feel, at various points, as though it is in tension with everything else here, because a great deal of what follows is an argument that you should know more, ask harder, and stop deferring to a system that is not organized around noticing you. Both are true. The system is not built to catch what it needs to catch, and you are the person best placed to catch it, and you are still not the person who should be adjusting a drug with a narrow therapeutic index on the basis of a chapter you read on a Tuesday.

What this book gives you is not autonomy over the dose. It is the ability to walk into a ten-minute appointment knowing which question is worth the ten minutes.

Before You Read Chapter 1.0

One piece of homework, and it takes about four minutes.

Write down every mood stabiliser you take. The dose. When you started it. And the date of your last blood test, if you can find it.

Most people cannot complete that list. If you cannot, that is not a criticism of you. It is the first finding of the book.

Chapter 1.0: Why Lithium Is Still First

The oldest drug in psychiatry is also the best one. Not the best tolerated. Not the most convenient. Not the one with the fewest blood tests, the friendliest side effect profile, or the biggest marketing budget, because it has never had a marketing budget at all. Lithium is an element. Nobody owns it. No company has ever had a reason to sell it to your doctor. And yet after seventy-five years of drug development, thousands of trials, and several generations of compounds designed by people who knew exactly what they were aiming at, lithium still sits at the top of every international guideline for the long-term treatment of bipolar disorder. That is not sentiment. That is the data.

1.1 What a Mood Stabiliser Actually Is

There is no agreed definition. That is the first thing worth knowing, and almost nobody says it out loud.

The phrase **mood stabiliser** entered common use in the 1990s, largely through pharmaceutical marketing, and it has never had a settled clinical meaning. The strictest version says a mood stabiliser must treat both poles of bipolar disorder, mania and depression, and prevent both from returning, without pushing the person into the opposite pole. Under that definition, almost nothing qualifies. Lithium comes closest. Everything else on the list fails at least one of the four tests.

The looser version, which is what most prescribers actually mean, is something like: a drug we use for the long haul in bipolar disorder that is not primarily an antipsychotic and not primarily an antidepressant. Under that definition, this book covers four: lithium, valproate, lamotrigine, and carbamazepine.

That vagueness matters to you for a practical reason. When your prescriber says "we'll start a mood stabiliser," they have told you almost nothing about what the drug will do. Lamotrigine and lithium are both mood stabilisers, and they do close to opposite jobs. Lamotrigine mostly holds the floor up. Lithium mostly holds the ceiling down, and does something to the floor too, though less reliably than anyone would like. If you have been on both and found them completely different experiences, that is because they are completely different drugs sharing a category name invented by a marketing department.

1.2 A Guess That Happened to Be Right

John Cade was an Australian psychiatrist working out of a disused kitchen at a repatriation hospital in Melbourne. In 1949 he published a paper reporting that lithium salts calmed patients in states of psychotic excitement. His reasoning for trying lithium in the first place was, by any modern standard, wrong. He had a theory about a toxin in the urine of manic patients, he was injecting guinea pigs, and he used lithium urate mainly because it was the most soluble urate salt available to him. The guinea pigs went placid. He tried it on ten patients. It worked.

It is worth being honest about this. One of the two or three most important discoveries in the history of psychiatric medicine came out of an experiment whose premise was mistaken, run on the wrong animal, for the wrong reason, by a man with no research funding and no laboratory.

What followed was not a triumphant adoption. Lithium was nearly lost. In the same period, lithium chloride had been marketed in the United States as a salt substitute for cardiac patients, who were not monitored, took it freely, and some of whom died. The compound acquired a reputation for danger that took two decades and a great deal of Scandinavian persistence to undo. Mogens Schou in Denmark ran the trials that established maintenance efficacy, and spent much of his career arguing with a field that had decided lithium was poison.

Both things were true, which is the part the field took twenty years to absorb. Lithium is poison at the wrong level. It is also the most effective long-term treatment psychiatry has. The entire architecture of monitoring described in this book exists to hold those two facts apart, and it exists because of what happened to the cardiac patients in 1949, not because of anything that happened to a psychiatric patient.

That history has a residue you may have encountered without recognizing it. Lithium prescribing has fallen steadily in the United States for thirty years while prescribing of newer agents has risen (Post, 2018). The decline does not track a decline in the evidence. The evidence got stronger. What fell away was the commercial reason to talk about it, and the willingness of prescribers to take on a drug that requires them to organize monitoring rather than write a script and move on. If you have been offered lithium, you have been offered it by someone who is prepared to do more work than the alternative required of them. That is worth knowing.

1.3 What It Does and What Nobody Knows

Here is the uncomfortable part. After seventy-five years, we do not know how lithium works.

We know a great deal about what it *does*. It inhibits an enzyme called glycogen synthase kinase-3 beta. It depletes inositol through inhibition of inositol monophosphatase. It shifts the balance of glutamate signaling, alters circadian gene expression, and increases levels of a protein called BDNF that is involved in keeping neurons alive and adaptable. Malhi and colleagues (2013) catalogued these pathways and reached the conclusion that most researchers reach: several of these are probably relevant, no single one is clearly the mechanism, and the honest position is that we have a list rather than an explanation.

Compare that to the story you were probably told. A chemical imbalance. Lithium corrects it. That story is tidy, it is what most leaflets imply, and it is not supported by anything.

Why does this matter to someone taking the tablet? Because the not-knowing has a consequence you will run into. Nobody can predict who will respond. There is no blood test, no scan, and no genetic panel that tells you in advance whether lithium is your drug. What we do know is that response clusters in families, that it is more likely in classic episodic bipolar I with clean recovery between episodes, and that the people who respond tend to respond *extremely* well, which is why Alda (2015) and others have argued that lithium response may mark out a distinct biological subgroup rather than a point on a spectrum. If lithium works for you, it may work for decades. The only way to find out is to take it and see, which is a genuinely unsatisfying thing to be told and also the truth.

1.4 Four Things People Get Wrong

The first is that lithium is a sedative. It is not. It does not work by flattening you, and if you feel flattened on lithium that is a side effect worth investigating rather than the drug doing its job. The confusion comes from Cade's original 1949 report, which described agitated patients becoming calm, and from the fact that lithium is often started during mania alongside something that genuinely is sedating. The lithium was not what made you sleep.

The second is that lithium levels tell you how well you are. They do not. A level tells you how much lithium is in your blood at the moment the needle went in. That is all it tells you. Chapter 2.0 takes this apart properly, because more damage is done by misunderstanding this one number than by almost anything else in this book.

The third is that a higher level means better protection. The relationship is not linear and it does not continue upward. The ISBD and IGSLI task force reviewed this specifically and concluded that the standard maintenance range sits around 0.60 to 0.80 mmol/L for most people, with some benefit from going higher in some patients and a clear tolerability cost for doing so (Nolen et al., 2019). Above the range, you are not buying more prevention. You are buying tremor, thirst, and eventually toxicity.

The fourth is the one that causes the most avoidable harm. People believe that if they feel well, the drug has finished its work. Lithium is not an antibiotic. There is no course. The wellness is the drug working, which is precisely why the wellness is not evidence that you can stop, and this is the single most circular and most frustrating fact in the whole of maintenance psychiatry.

1.5 The Thing That Justifies the Blood Tests

Every drug in this book prevents relapse to some degree. Only one of them appears to stop people dying.

Cipriani and colleagues (2013) pooled 48 randomized trials covering more than 6,600 participants and found that lithium reduced the number of deaths by suicide compared with placebo. Baldessarini's earlier meta-analytic work (2006) found roughly a fivefold reduction in suicides and attempts during long-term lithium treatment. The effect appears in mood disorders generally, not only bipolar. And, importantly, it does not track neatly with lithium's mood-episode prevention, which raises the possibility that the antisuicidal effect is a separate action of the drug rather than a downstream consequence of being less ill.

That last point is contested. Some of the trials were not designed to measure suicide as a primary outcome, the event rates are low, and the meta-analytic estimates carry wide intervals. Nobody should present this as settled to three decimal places.

But it is the strongest signal of its kind in psychiatric pharmacology, and no other mood stabiliser has produced anything comparable. That is the arithmetic behind the monitoring burden. Four blood tests a year is a real cost. It is a real cost measured against a real benefit, which is more than can be said for a lot of what gets prescribed.

The following account is a composite, with details changed for anonymity.

Kestrel had been on lithium for eleven years when she started asking to come off. Her argument was reasonable and she had thought it through. She had not had a manic episode since 2015. She had not been hospitalized since her twenties. She was, by every measure her psychiatrist used, well. She wanted to know why she was still taking a drug for a problem she no longer had, and she wanted to know why nobody could give her a straight answer.

Her psychiatrist gave her the standard reply about maintenance treatment, which Kestrel had heard before and found circular. You are well because of the drug. How do you know? Because you are well.

She was right that it's circular. This is the central epistemic problem of maintenance treatment and there is no clean way around it. You cannot run a controlled trial on one person's life. The absence of episodes is compatible with the drug working, with the illness having burned out, and with eleven years of luck.

What changed her thinking was not an argument. It was a number. Her psychiatrist showed her the discontinuation data: that relapse rates after stopping lithium are high, that the risk concentrates heavily in the first several months, and that rapid discontinuation appears worse than gradual. Kestrel had assumed stopping would return her to her pre-lithium baseline. It might not. It might return her to something worse, at a point in her life when she had far more to lose than she did at 24.

She stayed on it. She is not happy about it. Eleven years in, she still resents the tablet, and she takes it anyway, and both of those facts are allowed to be true at once.

1.6 What Lithium Is Not Good At

The following is a composite case; identifying details have been changed.

Background Merritt, 41, had been on lithium for six years following a bipolar I diagnosis in his early thirties. He was maintained at a level in the middle of the accepted therapeutic range. He had not had a manic episode since starting.

Presentation He attended a routine review reporting eight months of low mood, oversleeping, weight gain, and near-total loss of interest in work he had previously cared about. He was not suicidal. He described the state as "flat, not sad." He had raised it twice before and had been told his lithium level was fine.

Analysis His lithium level was fine. That was the problem, not the reassurance. Lithium's evidence base is far stronger for preventing mania than for treating or preventing bipolar depression. Miura and colleagues (2014) found in their network meta-analysis that maintenance agents differ substantially by pole, and lithium's advantage is clearest against the manic pole. A therapeutic lithium level does not rule out a depressive episode. It never did. But "your level is fine" gets heard as "there is nothing wrong," which is a different sentence entirely.

Two other explanations were live. His TSH had not been checked in fourteen months, and lithium-induced hypothyroidism produces exactly this picture. His weight gain could have been driving the low mood, or the low mood could have been driving the weight gain, and nothing in the notes distinguished them.

Intervention TSH was checked first, before any psychiatric change. It came back elevated. Thyroid replacement was started. Lamotrigine was added three months later when the mood had improved but not resolved.

Outcome At nine months he described himself as roughly two thirds better. He remained on lithium. He was still annoyed that the answer had taken eight months and two dismissed complaints to arrive at, which seems to me a proportionate response.

> **Teaching Point:** *A therapeutic lithium level tells you about lithium. It tells you nothing about the depressive pole.*
>
> **Teaching Point:** *Hypothyroidism and depression present identically and are distinguished by a blood test, not by clinical impression.*
>
> **Teaching Point:** *"Your level is fine" is a statement about a number. Patients hear it as a statement about them.*

1.7 The Throughline

Start here: lithium is first-line in every international guideline not because it is old and cheap, but because on the two things that matter most over a lifetime, preventing manic relapse and reducing death, nothing has beaten it. Build on that: the reason it demands blood tests is the same reason it works, which is that the gap between the dose that helps and the dose that harms is narrow enough to need measuring, and the measuring is the price of admission rather than an administrative failure. Then add this: none of that makes lithium a good drug for everything. It is weak against the depressive pole, it causes hypothyroidism that looks exactly like depression, and a therapeutic level answers one question only.

Put those three together and you get the shape of the rest of this book. Not "lithium is wonderful." Not "lithium is dangerous." Something more useful and less comfortable, which is that this is a drug with a genuinely favorable risk-benefit ratio that only stays favorable if somebody is paying attention, and the person best placed to pay attention is you.

Kestrel is still taking it. Merritt spent eight months depressed inside a therapeutic range. Neither of those facts is an argument against the drug. They are arguments for understanding it, which is a different thing, and the next chapter starts where that understanding has to start. Not with the tablet. With the test.

Chapter 2.0: What the Blood Test Measures

The form is usually yellow, or pink, or whatever color that particular lab has settled on. It has your name on it, a date of birth, a barcode, and a row of boxes with abbreviations in them. Somebody has ticked four or five. You handed it over at a desk, held out your arm, watched the tube fill, and went to work. The whole thing took nine minutes.

That form is the most important document in your treatment, and almost nobody who fills one in has been told what the ticked boxes are looking for. This chapter is about the boxes.

2.1 Why This Drug Needs Measuring

Most medications do not require blood tests. You take the dose, it does the thing, and the gap between a useful amount and a harmful amount is wide enough that nobody needs to check where in that gap you happen to be sitting.

Lithium has a **narrow therapeutic index**, which is the pharmacological term for a small gap between the dose that works and the dose that hurts you. For most people on maintenance treatment, the useful range sits somewhere around 0.60 to 0.80 mmol/L (Nolen et al., 2019). Toxicity becomes a serious concern above 1.5 mmol/L, and people have been badly hurt at 2.0. That is a factor of about two and a half between working and dangerous. For comparison, you could take five times the standard dose of most antidepressants and be uncomfortable rather than in an intensive care unit.

The gap is narrow, and it moves. It moves when you sweat, when you vomit, when you start a blood pressure tablet, when you cut salt out of your diet, when you get dehydrated on a hot day. Chapter 7.0 covers the moving. This chapter covers the measuring.

One number is worth sitting with. Lithium is cleared almost entirely by your kidneys, and it is handled by them in more or less the same way as sodium. Your kidneys cannot tell the two apart. That single fact of chemistry explains nearly everything strange about this drug: why dehydration raises your level, why a low-salt diet raises your level, why a diuretic that makes you excrete sodium can make you retain lithium, why a stomach bug is a lithium event, and why an August heatwave is a medical circumstance for you and not for the person next to you. Nothing about lithium is arbitrary once you know that it is impersonating salt.

There is a second reason for the tests, and it is the one people forget. The serum lithium level is only one of the boxes. The others are not checking the drug. They are checking you, specifically your thyroid, your kidneys, and your parathyroid glands, all of which lithium can affect over years in ways that produce no symptoms until they produce a great many.

2.2 The Twelve Hour Rule

Here is the single most useful fact in this book.

A lithium level means nothing unless the blood was drawn approximately twelve hours after your last dose. Not eight. Not four. Twelve, give or take about an hour.

This is not a technicality. Lithium concentration in your blood rises after you swallow the tablet, peaks somewhere in the following one to three hours depending on the formulation, and then falls. If you sample during the peak, you get a high number that reflects nothing about your maintenance state. If you sample at eighteen hours, you get a low number for the same reason. The whole system of reference ranges you will ever be measured against was built on twelve-hour post-dose samples (Amdisen, 1977). Every published range, every guideline threshold, every number in this book assumes it.

There is a second timing fact that follows from the first, and it catches people out at the pharmacy counter rather than the phlebotomy chair. Lithium brands are not interchangeable. Lithium carbonate and lithium citrate contain different amounts of lithium, and even among carbonate products the release characteristics differ enough that a swap changes your level. If your usual brand is out of stock and a well-meaning pharmacist offers you a different one, that is not a like-for-like substitution. It is a dose change that requires a level check. Prescriptions for lithium are written by brand for exactly this reason, and if yours has quietly changed, your next level is not comparable to your last one.

The following worked example uses a composite case.

Hollis took her lithium at 10 p.m., which suited her because it was when she brushed her teeth. Her blood test appointment was offered at 9 a.m., which suited the surgery because that was when the phlebotomist started.

Step 1: What the numbers said Her level came back at 0.9 mmol/L. Her prescriber, seeing a level at the top of the range in a patient reporting a fine tremor, reduced her dose from 800 mg to 600 mg.

Step 2: What was actually measured The sample was drawn eleven hours after her dose. That is close enough to twelve to be usable. So far, nothing has gone wrong.

Step 3: Where it broke Three months later the surgery moved her review to a 2 p.m. slot. Sixteen hours post-dose. The level came back at 0.5 mmol/L, which read as subtherapeutic. Her dose went back up to 800 mg. Nobody recorded the sampling time on either occasion, because the form has no box for it.

The complicating moment The obvious reading is that Hollis was under-treated and the dose correction was right. It was not. She had been at a perfectly reasonable level throughout, sampled at three different points on the same curve, and had her dose moved twice for no clinical reason. The second increase produced a genuine rise in tremor, which she attributed to stress at work, and which resolved when the timing error was eventually spotted.

Step 4: What fixed it Hollis started writing the time of her last dose on the top of the request form in pen. Not because anyone asked her to. Because nobody else was going to.

What this worked example shows The system has no reliable mechanism for capturing sampling time, and the reference range is meaningless without it. Which means the person who has to hold that information is the person whose dose depends on it.

2.3 What Each Box Is Ruling Out

Serum lithium. How much lithium is in your blood twelve hours after your dose. It answers one question: is your dose in the range? It does not answer whether you are well, whether the drug is working, or whether you are about to relapse.

TSH, thyroid stimulating hormone. Lithium interferes with the thyroid gland's ability to release hormone. Somewhere between 6 and 20 percent of people on long-term lithium develop hypothyroidism, and it is more common in women (Shine et al., 2015). A rising TSH means the pituitary is shouting at a thyroid that isn't responding. The symptoms of that, tiredness, weight gain, low mood, slowness of thought, are indistinguishable from depression by clinical impression alone, which is exactly what happened to Merritt in Chapter 1.0. This box exists because you cannot tell the difference by how you feel.

Creatinine and eGFR. Kidney function. Creatinine is a waste product your kidneys clear; eGFR is a calculated estimate of how fast they are clearing it. The number matters less than the direction. One eGFR of 72 tells you very little. Five eGFRs over six years tell you a great deal. Chapter 9.0 is about what those five numbers mean and what they do not.

Calcium. This is the one that surprises people, and it is on the schedule for a real reason. Long-term lithium is associated with hyperparathyroidism and raised blood calcium. The presentation is vague, tiredness, low mood, constipation, thirst, and it gets attributed to the illness or to the lithium's more famous side effects for years. Shine and colleagues (2015), reviewing laboratory data on nearly 5,000 patients, found the association with raised calcium was actually clearer than some of the renal findings.

Weight and BMI. Not a blood test, but it belongs on the same schedule, for reasons Chapter 11.0 covers.

Two things are missing from that list that people expect to find. There is no test for whether lithium is working. There is also no test that predicts whether it will. Both absences frustrate patients enormously, and both are honest. What the panel gives you is a safety picture and a dose picture. The efficacy picture is assembled from your life, over years, by you and the people who know you, which is one of the reasons Chapter 13.0 exists.

For valproate and carbamazepine the box list is different: full blood count and liver function tests, and for carbamazepine, sodium. Their chapters cover why.

2.4 How Often and Why That Number Slips

The standard in the United Kingdom, set out in NICE guideline CG185, is every six months for lithium level, thyroid function, renal function, and calcium, with more frequent testing for older adults, anyone on an interacting medication, anyone with existing renal, thyroid, or electrolyte concerns, and anyone whose dose has recently changed. Levels are checked weekly after initiation or a dose change until stable. International practice varies but the shape is similar (Malhi et al., 2017).

That is the standard. Practice is another matter, and the literature on this is not flattering. Collins and colleagues (2010) audited lithium monitoring across UK mental health trusts and found substantial shortfalls against the standard. Paton and colleagues (2013) ran a quality improvement program and demonstrated that the shortfalls were improvable, which is another way of saying they were real. A National Patient Safety Agency alert in 2009 was issued specifically because monitoring failures were producing harm. Surveys of international practice find the same pattern in other countries (Nederlof et al., 2018).

Kirkham and colleagues (2014) added a finding that sharpens why this matters. Reviewing a monitoring database, they found that a single lithium level above 1.0 mmol/L was followed by an acute decline in eGFR. One episode. Not years of gentle exposure. That is an argument for catching a high level early rather than at the next scheduled six-month appointment, and it is an argument for taking a single out-of-range result seriously rather than filing it as a blip.

Nobody is being negligent on purpose. Lithium monitoring falls between primary care and specialist services in most systems, and things that fall between two services fall. The psychiatrist assumes the GP is doing the bloods. The GP assumes the psychiatrist is reviewing them. The result gets filed as normal by whoever opens it, which is often neither of them, and a slow drift in a calcium level over four years is precisely the kind of thing that no single person in that arrangement is looking at. The practical consequence for you is uncomfortable and worth stating plainly: the person most reliably positioned to notice that your calcium has not been checked in two years is you.

2.5 When the Number Is Wrong

The following account is a composite, with details changed for anonymity.

Arden had been on lithium for nine years and had never had a level outside the range. He was, in his own description, a boring patient. Then a level came back at 1.4 mmol/L.

His prescriber's first move was the right one, which was to ask questions before changing anything. Had he changed the dose? No. Had he doubled up after a missed dose? No. Any new medication? He said no.

The level was repeated four days later and came back at 1.35 mmol/L. At that point the working assumption became that something had genuinely changed, and the dose was cut.

What had changed was that Arden's GP had started him on ramipril for blood pressure six weeks earlier. He had not mentioned it because, in his words, it was not a psychiatric medication. ACE inhibitors reduce lithium clearance. Nobody had asked the question in a form that would have got the right answer, because "any new medication" gets heard as "any new medication from a psychiatrist."

The recovery was straightforward once the cause was identified. The lithium dose was adjusted, the ramipril continued, and the monitoring interval was shortened for three months while the new equilibrium settled.

What is worth noticing is where the failure sat. Not in the lab. Not in the level, which was accurate. In the question. Arden answered honestly. He was asked the wrong thing.

> **Teaching Point:** *A single abnormal level should be repeated before it is acted on, unless the person is unwell.*

> **Teaching Point:** *"Any new medication" is a question that reliably fails. "What is in your bathroom cabinet, including things from your GP and things from a pharmacy shelf" is a question that works.*

2.6 Putting It to Work

The practical upshot is smaller than the chapter made it sound, and it comes down to four things you can start doing at your next appointment.

Write the time of your last dose on the form. Every time. If the form has nowhere to write it, write it in the margin. This costs you four seconds and it is the difference between a number that means something and a number that means nothing.

Keep the results yourself. Not the interpretation, the actual numbers, in one place, with dates. Appendix B is set up for this. The reason is not distrust of your clinicians. It is that you are likely to outlast several of them, and the trend across a decade is the clinically interesting object, and no single practitioner in your care will ever have seen the whole of it.

Know your four boxes: lithium, thyroid, kidney, calcium. When you attend for bloods, ask which are being done. If calcium has not been checked in more than a year, ask why. This is not a confrontation. Most of the time the answer will be that it fell off the form, and the fix is that you noticed.

And separate the two sentences that get conflated in every appointment you will ever have. "Your level is fine" means the dose is in range. "You are fine" is a different claim, requiring different evidence, and the person best placed to supply that evidence is sitting in the chair rather than reading the screen.

Chapter 3.0 moves to a drug with a different problem entirely. Lamotrigine needs no blood levels at all. What it needs is your attention for eight weeks.

Chapter 3.0: Lamotrigine and the Rash Question

The number everybody knows about lamotrigine is three in 1,000. It appears in the boxed warning, and it is the figure that gets quoted to patients starting the drug for bipolar disorder. It is also not their number. Three in 1,000 is the rate of serious rash in adults taking lamotrigine as add-on therapy for epilepsy. In the trials of lamotrigine in mood disorders, the rate was closer to one in 1,000, and in the controlled trials Calabrese and colleagues (2002) reviewed, not a single patient on lamotrigine had a serious rash. Meanwhile about eight in 100 got a harmless one. The famous number belongs to a different drug indication in a different population, and on the night a rash actually appears, standing in your bathroom at 11 p.m. with your shirt off, none of the three figures tells you which kind you have. Nobody can. Not you, not a telephone triage nurse, and in the first hours often not a dermatologist either. That gap between a reassuring statistic and a useless one, at the moment you actually need it, is what this chapter is about.

3.1 The Problem Nobody Solved Cleanly

Lamotrigine is the best drug in this book for the pole that hurts people most.

Bipolar depression accounts for the great majority of time spent unwell in bipolar disorder. It is what wrecks careers and marriages, and it is what kills people. Lithium is only modestly effective against it. Antidepressants are contentious and may destabilize. Lamotrigine, in the maintenance trials, delayed the time to a depressive episode in a way nothing else in the class reliably matched (Bowden et al., 2003; Goodwin et al., 2004). It also does not cause weight gain, does not require blood levels, does not touch the thyroid, and does not threaten the kidney. Read that list back. It is close to the ideal drug.

It has one problem. Sometimes it strips your skin off.

Stevens-Johnson syndrome and its more severe form, **toxic epidermal necrolysis**, are immune reactions in which the epidermis detaches from the layer beneath it, starting typically at the mucous membranes, the mouth, the eyes, the genitals, and spreading. They are treated in burns units. Mortality in the severe form runs above 30 percent. They are rare. They are also the reason lamotrigine carries a boxed warning and the reason your starter pack is a piece of cardboard with the doses printed on it like a calendar.

So the field had a problem with a shape. The best available drug for the worst pole of the illness carried a rare but catastrophic risk that appeared unpredictable, and the risk sat at the beginning of treatment, before anyone had received any benefit at all. A patient who stops in week five has taken all of the risk and none of the reward.

3.2 What Did Not Work

The first response was to look for who was vulnerable. If the reaction could be predicted, it could be avoided.

That search has been only partly successful, and it is worth understanding why, because the failure explains your starter pack. Hirsch and colleagues (2006) examined predictors of lamotrigine rash and found the signal weaker and messier than hoped. A personal history of rash on another antiepileptic raises risk, and there is meaningful cross-reactivity between aromatic antiepileptics, so someone who reacted to carbamazepine is more likely to react to lamotrigine (Wang et al., 2010). Younger age raises it. Concomitant valproate raises it substantially. Beyond that, the ability to look at a given adult and say "you are the one" essentially does not exist.

Pharmacogenetics helped for a different drug. HLA-B*1502 predicts carbamazepine-induced Stevens-Johnson syndrome strongly enough in some ancestries that testing changed practice, which Chapter 5.0 covers. For lamotrigine, the HLA associations are real but weaker and less consistent across populations, and they have not translated into a test that would let you skip the vigilance (Mullan et al., 2019). Epidemiological work by Mockenhaupt and colleagues (2005) and later by Frey and colleagues (2017) put the absolute risk in new users into perspective, which is useful for policy and cold comfort at 11 p.m.

Screening for the vulnerable person did not work. So the field stopped trying to find the person and went after the exposure instead.

3.3 The Pivot That Actually Worked

The insight was almost embarrassingly simple. The immune reaction seems to depend not just on the drug but on how fast the body meets it. Go slowly enough, and the reaction largely does not happen.

The dose schedule you have been given, which feels like bureaucratic caution, is the intervention. Twenty-five milligrams for two weeks. Fifty for two weeks. Then stepwise upward. It takes five or six weeks to reach a dose that does anything at all, which is a genuinely cruel thing to ask of a depressed person, and it is the single measure that made this drug usable. When manufacturers introduced the slow titration and the accompanying guidance, rates of serious rash in trials fell substantially (Guberman et al., 1999; Messenheimer et al., 1998). Calabrese and colleagues (2002) went looking for the damage across 12 multicenter mood disorder trials and largely did not find it. In the controlled trials, benign rash occurred in 8.3 percent of patients on lamotrigine against 6.4 percent on placebo, a difference of under two percentage points. Serious rash occurred in zero percent of lamotrigine patients. The only serious rash in the controlled setting was in someone taking placebo. In the open-label trials, where 13.1 percent had a rash of some kind, there were two serious cases, and one mild Stevens-Johnson syndrome that did not require hospitalization. Across the whole review, no cases of toxic epidermal necrolysis in any setting.

The manufacturer's own labeling puts the mood disorder figures at 0.08 percent for lamotrigine as initial monotherapy and 0.13 percent as adjunctive therapy. Call it one in 1,000. The 0.3 percent in the boxed warning is the epilepsy adjunctive figure, and the 0.8 percent alongside it is for children. Those numbers are real and they are not yours, and nobody points this out, which is why a drug whose serious rash rate in the trials that actually apply to you was close to nil is one of the most feared prescriptions in psychiatry.

Three consequences follow, and they are the whole practical content of this chapter.

The slowness is not negotiable and it is not caution. It is the mechanism. Speeding up the titration because you feel awful and want it to work faster is not impatience, it is a dose escalation of the specific variable that drives the risk.

Missing doses is a titration problem. If you stop lamotrigine for around five days or more, your tolerance is treated as lost and you restart the climb from the beginning. This is enraging and it is real. Doubling up to catch up is worse than the gap you were trying to fix.

Valproate changes the arithmetic completely. Valproate inhibits the enzyme that clears lamotrigine and can roughly double its concentration. If you are on both, your lamotrigine dose is typically halved and the climb is slower still. Somebody adding valproate to established lamotrigine without adjusting the lamotrigine is making a serious error.

3.4 The Window and the Red Flags

Nearly every serious lamotrigine rash appears between weeks two and eight of treatment. That is one of the most useful facts in this book, because it means the vigilance has an end date. You are not signing up to inspect yourself for the rest of your life. You are signing up for about six weeks.

Within that window, the features that escalate a rash from a nuisance to an emergency are not subtle once you know them. Fever. Involvement of the mouth, the eyes, the throat, or the genitals. Blistering. Skin that hurts rather than itches. Swollen glands. Feeling systemically ill, the way flu feels ill, rather than locally irritated. Rash on the face and upper trunk rather than the shins. Any of these, on lamotrigine, in the first two months, is a stop-the-drug-and-be-seen-today event.

Absent all of those, a mild itchy rash is more likely to be heat, laundry detergent, or one of the eight in 100 benign eruptions, which outnumber the serious ones by something on the order of 60 to one on the mood disorder figures. Which does not mean ignore it. It means call rather than panic, and take a photograph with the date on it, because rashes change faster than appointments arrive.

One more thing belongs in the window, and it is the reason Chapter 6.0 exists. If you are already on lamotrigine and somebody adds valproate, the window reopens. Your lamotrigine level will rise even though your lamotrigine dose has not changed, and you are back in the risk period without having done anything. Duan and colleagues (2023) reported a case of exactly this shape in an adolescent treated with both, who developed a generalized rash with swollen lymph nodes twelve days in and improved after the valproate was stopped and steroids were started. The lamotrigine was not the villain there. The combination was, and the point at which the combination began was the point at which vigilance should have restarted.

There is also a question people ask and rarely get answered honestly, which is what lamotrigine does apart from not causing a rash. The answer is: less than the marketing suggests and more than nothing. It prevents depressive episodes. It does not prevent mania, or not to any useful degree, which is why a person with bipolar I who is prone to mania is usually on lamotrigine plus something else rather than lamotrigine alone. Presenting it as a mood stabiliser in the full sense, holding both poles, oversells it. It holds one. The other has to be held by something.

The following are composite cases.

Case A Fable started lamotrigine in March. In week six she developed an itchy pink rash across her forearms and shins after a weekend in the garden. She photographed it, phoned the duty line, and described it. No fever. No mouth or eye involvement. Nothing on her trunk. She was seen the following morning, the rash was assessed as benign, and she was advised to continue with a low threshold for calling again. It faded over nine days. She reached her target dose in week eight and had her first genuinely level summer in six years.

Case B Linden started lamotrigine in the same month. In week three she developed a rash on her chest and neck, felt achy, and thought she had picked up a virus. She had a temperature of 38.1 and a sore throat, which she attributed to the virus. She waited four days. By the time she attended, she had lesions inside her mouth.

The contrast is not about how bad each rash looked, and this is where intuition fails people. Fable's rash was more visible and more uncomfortable. Linden's began as something she could easily dismiss. What distinguished them was fever plus mucosal involvement plus systemic illness, three features that were present in one case and absent in the other, and which are checkable in about fifteen seconds by anyone who knows to check.

What both cases had in common was that the decision took minutes rather than days. That is the design goal. You are not being asked to become a dermatologist. You are being asked to run a three-item check and then hand the problem to someone else, quickly, with a photograph.

3.5 Where the Slow Climb Costs Something

The titration schedule solved the rash problem by transferring the cost somewhere else. That transfer is real and it is under-acknowledged.

The following account is a composite, with details changed for anonymity.

Briar was severely depressed when lamotrigine was started. Not mildly. She was sleeping fourteen hours, had stopped answering her phone, and had been signed off work for a month. Her psychiatrist explained the schedule: 25 mg, then 50, then upward, with a therapeutic dose somewhere around week six or seven.

Briar did the arithmetic in the room and said what a lot of people think and do not say, which was that six weeks was a long time to ask someone in her state to wait for a drug to start.

She was right. This is the honest weakness of lamotrigine and it does not get said often enough. It is a maintenance drug wearing the clothes of a treatment. Geddes et al. (2009), reanalyzing individual patient data across five randomized trials, found the acute antidepressant effect of lamotrigine to be statistically real but modest, and concentrated in more severely depressed patients.

Modest and slow is a difficult sell to someone who cannot get off the sofa.

What her psychiatrist did was not to argue with the timeline but to stop pretending the timeline was fine. Something else was added to cover the interval. The lamotrigine kept climbing underneath it. The plan named lamotrigine as the thing that would still be working in two years, not the thing that would help in two weeks.

Briar reached 200 mg in week eight and did not get a rash. She also did not experience a dramatic lift. What she reported at twelve months was that she had not had a bad winter, which is the kind of unspectacular outcome this drug produces and the kind that is almost impossible to feel grateful for in week three.

> **Teaching Point:** *The titration schedule buys safety with time, and the time is paid for by someone who is unwell.*
>
> **Teaching Point:** *Lamotrigine's honest indication is prevention. Presenting it as an acute treatment sets up a disappointment that reads to the patient as failure.*

3.6 What Earns Its Place

Fable is the reason this chapter exists rather than a warning label. She had the rash that more than nine in 10 people never get, in the window when it matters, and she handled it in about four minutes: look, photograph, check three things, phone. She was not brave and she was not lucky. She had been told what to look at, which is the entire intervention.

Linden had been told too. What she had not been told was that fever counted, so the one feature that should have moved her did the opposite, because a temperature and a sore throat in week three read to her as evidence that it was a virus rather than the drug. That is not a failure of vigilance. It is a failure of the briefing.

So what earns its place here is narrow. Not "watch for a rash," which is what the leaflet says and which produces either nightly inspection or nothing. Three features, one window. Fever, mucous membranes, feeling ill all over. Weeks two to eight. Everything else in this chapter is scaffolding around those two lines, and if you remember nothing else from it, remember the fever, because it is the one that gets misread as innocent.

The rest of the drug is close to a gift. No levels, no thyroid, no kidney, no weight, and a genuine effect on the pole that does the most damage. You pay for it once, at the start, with six weeks of attention. That is a good trade, and it is only a good trade if you know what you are attending to.

Chapter 4.0 turns to the drug where the trade went the other way, and where the whole regulatory apparatus of a country eventually decided the price was too high.

Chapter 4.0: Valproate and the Rules

In 1963, in a laboratory in Grenoble, a chemist needed to dissolve some compounds he wanted to test for anticonvulsant activity. He reached for a solvent that had been sitting on chemistry shelves since 1882, when a man named Burton first synthesized it, and which had never done anything more interesting than dissolve things. Every compound he dissolved in it turned out to be an anticonvulsant. Every single one. It took the group a while to work out that the compounds were irrelevant and the solvent was the drug (Meunier et al., 1963). Valproic acid had been sitting in plain view for eighty-one years, and it was found because somebody used it to wash the glassware.

4.1 A Drug Found by Accident and Kept on Purpose

Accidental discovery is not a mark against a drug. Lithium's origin story is no better and penicillin's is worse. What matters is what happened next, and what happened next was that valproate turned out to be genuinely, unusually good.

It works in epilepsy across seizure types where other agents are narrow. In psychiatry, Bowden and colleagues (1994) established in a randomized comparison against lithium and placebo that divalproex was effective in acute mania, and it worked faster than lithium did. It does not need a twelve-hour trough taken with the precision described in Chapter 2.0. It does not damage kidneys. It can be loaded, meaning a person in an acute manic episode can be brought to a therapeutic dose in days rather than weeks, which in an inpatient unit at 2 a.m. is worth a great deal.

For about thirty years, valproate was the sensible choice. It became one of the most prescribed drugs in psychiatry and neurology in the world. If you are over 40 and have bipolar disorder, there is a fair chance you have taken it, and a fair chance it worked.

That is the part of the story that gets left out of the current conversation, and leaving it out is a mistake, because it makes the last decade look like the correction of an obvious error. It was not obvious. It was a good drug with a hidden cost, and the cost took a very long time to be counted.

4.2 What the Cost Turned Out to Be

The first signal appeared in 1982. Robert and Guibaud published a short report in The Lancet linking maternal valproic acid to neural tube defects, specifically spina bifida. Two years later, DiLiberti and colleagues (1984) described a recognizable pattern of facial features and malformations in children exposed in utero and gave it a name: fetal valproate syndrome.

So the physical malformation risk has been known since roughly 1982. Read that date again. The structural risk was in the literature before a large proportion of the people currently taking valproate were born.

The scale, as it was eventually pinned down, is this. Around three to five percent of pregnancies exposed to valproate result in a neural tube defect, against a background rate of well under one percent. The overall major congenital malformation rate is higher still and dose-dependent; the MHRA's own public figure, the one printed on the patient materials, is roughly one in nine. Tomson and colleagues (2018), reporting the EURAP registry across eight antiepileptic drugs, found valproate carried the highest malformation risk of the group, and that risk rose steeply with dose. Carbamazepine sat well below it. Lamotrigine sat lowest.

The second signal took another twenty years and it is the larger one.

Malformations are visible at birth. Cognitive and developmental effects are not, and you cannot detect them without following exposed children for years. Meador and colleagues (2013), in the NEAD study, followed children to age six and found valproate-exposed children had significantly lower IQ than those exposed to other antiepileptics, with a dose relationship. Christensen and colleagues (2013), using Danish national registry data, found an increased risk of autism spectrum disorder and childhood autism after prenatal valproate exposure. Bromley and colleagues (2013) found a raised prevalence of neurodevelopmental disorders in exposed children.

Roughly 30 to 40 percent of children exposed to valproate in utero have some form of developmental disorder, or three to four in every 10, which is how the MHRA now phrases it to patients. That figure, not the neural tube defects, is what changed the regulatory position, and it did not become clear until around 2013.

4.3 The Turning Point Was Not a Study

By 2014 the evidence was settled enough. The prescribing did not settle with it.

What actually moved the system was not a paper. It was the families. In the United Kingdom, an organized campaign by affected families, working over years, forced a review that most of the medical establishment did not want. Baroness Cumberlege's Independent Medicines and Medical Devices Safety Review reported in 2020 under the title First Do No Harm. It examined valproate alongside two other interventions and concluded that patients had been harmed, that they had been dismissed when they reported it, and that the system had been slow, defensive, and unwilling to hear them.

That is a finding about institutions, not about pharmacology. It is also the reason your prescriber's behavior around this drug looks the way it does. The forms, the annual reviews, the two signatures: none of that came out of a pharmacology department. It came out of a public reckoning in which the regulator was told, in writing, that it had failed.

The MHRA had introduced a Pregnancy Prevention Programme in 2018, requiring that valproate not be used in any woman or girl able to have children unless the conditions of that programme were met. Data suggested it was working, partially. Prescriptions to women aged 14 to 45 in England fell. The number of pregnant women prescribed valproate in a six-month window fell from 68 in 2018 to 17 by early 2022. Better. Not zero. In 2023 the Commission on Human Medicines reviewed the position and concluded that the existing requirements were not being consistently followed, and a National Patient Safety Alert instructed organizations to prepare for something considerably firmer.

4.4 Where the Rules Stand Now

What follows is dated deliberately, because this is the fastest-moving content in this book and you should be able to tell how old it is.

From 31 January 2024. Valproate must not be started in any new patient under 55, male or female, unless two specialists independently consider and document that there is no other effective or tolerated treatment, or that the reproductive risks do not apply. Women and girls already taking it are reviewed at their next annual specialist review using a revised Annual Risk Acknowledgement Form. Two specialists sign off continuation at that first annual review; at subsequent reviews, one specialist, in consultation with the patient.

From September 2024. The MHRA advised that men taking valproate, and their female partners, should use effective contraception during treatment and for three months after stopping. The advice followed a retrospective observational study suggesting a possible increased risk of neurodevelopmental disorders in children born to men taking valproate in the three months before conception.

From 13 February 2025. Following further review by the Commission on Human Medicines, the position was revised. Dual specialist review remains in place for anyone initiating valproate under 55, male or female. It is no longer required for men already taking it. Men already on valproate should be asked at their next review whether they plan to start a family within the next year, and if so, referred to discuss alternatives. The MHRA issued three infographics at the same time, which is what a regulator does when it has worked out that nobody can follow the rules it wrote.

From June 2025. The safety and educational materials were updated again, in line with the existing regulatory position and in response to stakeholder feedback rather than to any new restriction. The revised materials carry two things worth knowing: the precautionary paternal advice, and a risk that had not previously featured in this account, which is lower weight at birth for gestational age in children exposed to valproate during pregnancy.

Three pathways, then. Female under 55, initiating or continuing: the Pregnancy Prevention Programme, highly effective contraception, an Annual Risk Acknowledgement Form, and annual specialist review. Male under 55, already taking it: no dual review, the contraception advice, and a question about family plans at each review. Anyone initiating under 55, either sex: two specialists, independently, documented.

4.5 The Part Where This Gets Uncomfortable

The male measures were strongly criticized, and you are entitled to know that.

An evidence review conducted around the time of the September 2024 advice concluded that there was no clear evidence for an adverse impact of paternal antiseizure medication use on offspring outcomes. Specialists argued, publicly, that the risks of moving men onto less effective medication, including breakthrough seizures, hospitalization, and death, outweighed a paternal risk they considered unlikely. The February 2025 revision, which removed the dual review requirement for men already taking valproate, is best read as a partial acknowledgement that the criticism landed.

This is the honest position. The maternal evidence is overwhelming and has been for a decade. The paternal evidence is one retrospective observational signal, contested by people with no obvious axe to grind, and the regulatory response to it has already been revised once in under six months.

If you are a man on valproate who was told in 2024 that you needed two specialists and told in 2025 that you did not, the inconsistency was real and your clinician was not incompetent. You were living inside a regulator adjusting its position in real time on thin evidence, in the shadow of a public inquiry that had recently told it that it acted too slowly last time. That is the actual explanation, and no one is going to give it to you in a ten-minute appointment.

The following account is a composite, with details changed for anonymity.

Vesper had taken valproate for nine years. She had a bipolar I diagnosis, two prior hospital admissions, both before valproate, and none since. She was 38. She had been sterilized at 33 and had no intention of becoming pregnant under any circumstances.

Her annual review, the first under the revised process, went badly. She experienced the Risk Acknowledgement Form as an accusation. She had said, every year for nine years, that pregnancy was not a possibility for her, and every year the form came back. She began the appointment defensive and left it angry, and her clinician recorded in the notes that she had been resistant to the discussion.

The word resistant is doing a great deal of work in that sentence, and it is doing it in the wrong direction.

What Vesper had not been told was that the framework contains an explicit provision for exactly her situation: initiation and continuation are permitted where there are compelling reasons that the reproductive risks do not apply. She was not being accused of anything. She was being processed through a form designed for a population she was not a member of, by a clinician who had not read her far enough to say so.

The second appointment, six weeks later with a different specialist, took eleven minutes. He read the surgical history, said the sentence about compelling reasons out loud, signed the form, and moved on to how she was actually doing. Nothing pharmacological changed. What changed was that somebody named the category she was in.

> **Teaching Point:** *The regulatory framework contains exemptions. Patients are rarely told the exemptions exist.*
>
> **Teaching Point:** *"Resistant to the discussion" is often a note about the discussion, not the patient.*

The following is a composite case; identifying details have been changed.

Background Pax, 29, had bipolar I disorder with a history of severe manic episodes requiring admission. He had trialed lithium (stopped for tremor and a level that would not stabilize), quetiapine (stopped for weight and sedation), and aripiprazole (stopped for akathisia). Valproate had been started in 2021 and had held him well for three years.

Presentation He attended in late 2024 having received a letter about the new advice for men. He was in a two-year relationship. They had discussed children, without a timeline. He arrived with two questions: was he going to be taken off the drug, and had he already done something irreversible.

Analysis Neither question had a clean answer, and pretending otherwise would have been the easier and worse option. The paternal signal was one retrospective observational study. An evidence review had found no clear effect of paternal antiseizure medication on offspring outcomes. The precautionary advice was real; the evidence beneath it was thin. As of the February 2025 revision, Pax, already established on valproate, did not require dual specialist review. He did require the family-plans question, and he had just answered it in a way that triggered the referral.

His treatment history was the harder problem. Three prior agents had failed for tolerability rather than efficacy, which narrows the alternatives considerably and makes the phrase "no other effective or tolerated treatment" a description of his actual life rather than a box.

Intervention The clinician did three things. Named the evidence honestly, including its weakness. Confirmed that no change was being forced. And started the alternatives conversation on a twelve-month horizon rather than a six-week one, because Pax was not planning conception imminently and a rushed switch carried a relapse risk that was not hypothetical for a man with two prior admissions.

Outcome At six months Pax remained on valproate. A lamotrigine cross-titration had been started and then paused when his partner's plans changed. He described the conversation, not the outcome, as the useful part.

> **Teaching Point:** *"No other effective or tolerated treatment" is a clinical description for some people, not a form of words.*
>
> **Teaching Point:** *A precautionary rule with weak evidence still requires a real conversation. It does not require a rushed switch.*
>
> **Teaching Point:** *Failure for tolerability is not the same as failure for efficacy, and it constrains the alternatives differently.*

4.6 The Honest Summary

Four things are settled and are not going to move.

Valproate in pregnancy causes physical malformations in around three to five percent of exposures, and that has been known since the early 1980s. Valproate in pregnancy causes neurodevelopmental harm in roughly 30 to 40 percent of exposed children, and that has been reasonably clear since about 2013. The system knew both of these and kept prescribing anyway, which is what the Cumberlege review found and said. And valproate is, for some people, an effective drug that nothing else has replaced, which is why it has been restricted rather than withdrawn.

Three things are not settled.

Whether the paternal risk is real at all. One observational signal, an evidence review finding no clear effect, a precautionary rule, and a revision within six months. That is a system reasoning in public with insufficient data, and the honest description is that nobody knows yet.

Whether the two-specialist requirement helps patients or mostly protects institutions. It is defensible either way and it has not been evaluated.

And whether the pendulum has swung too far for men, and for women who cannot become pregnant, both of whom are now inside a framework built for a risk that does not apply to them, and both of whom are frequently not told that the framework says so.

What you can do with that is narrow but real. Find out which of the three pathways you are on. If reproductive risk genuinely does not apply to you, say the words compelling reasons at your next review, because they are in the framework and they are yours to use. If you are a man being asked about contraception, you are entitled to know the evidence for that request is thin and was recently revised.

Chapter 5.0 turns to the last of the four, and to a drug with the strangest property of any in this book. It changes while you take it.

Chapter 5.0: The Drug That Changes Itself

You take the same tablet every day and you expect the same thing to happen. That assumption is so basic that it does not feel like an assumption. The dose on the box is the dose. Two hundred milligrams on Monday is two hundred milligrams in March. Your body is the constant, the tablet is the variable, and if the drug stops working then either the illness got worse or the drug was never right for you.

Carbamazepine breaks that. It is the one drug in this book that teaches your body to get rid of it. The tablet does not change. Your capacity to destroy it does, over about three to five weeks, until the dose that was working is delivering roughly half of what it delivered at the start. Nothing has gone wrong. The drug is doing exactly what carbamazepine does, and almost nobody taking it has been told.

5.1 The Concept Nobody Explains

Autoinduction is the property of a drug that increases the activity of the enzymes responsible for clearing it. Carbamazepine is cleared mainly by an enzyme in the liver called CYP3A4. Carbamazepine also switches CYP3A4 production up. So the longer you take it, the more efficiently you dispose of it, and the same tablet produces a lower blood level week by week until the system reaches a new equilibrium.

Bertilsson and colleagues (1980) demonstrated this directly using stable isotope tracing, following on from earlier kinetic work by Eichelbaum and colleagues (1975) showing that single-dose and multiple-dose behavior of carbamazepine were not the same thing. The half-life of a first dose is somewhere around 25 to 35 hours. After a few weeks of regular dosing, it falls to something closer to 12 to 17 hours. The drug has roughly doubled its own clearance.

The process is largely complete by around week three to five. It then stops. It is not a slide into eventual uselessness, and this matters, because the natural reading when your medication stops working is that it will keep on not working.

Here is what this looks like from inside your life. Week one on carbamazepine: you feel a bit unsteady, a bit sedated, possibly slightly nauseated. Week three: those have eased and something is starting to settle. Week five: the settling has come undone. You are irritable again, or the sleep has gone, or the edge is back. You conclude, reasonably, that the drug worked for a fortnight and then failed. You may not report it, because a drug that works for a fortnight and then fails sounds like a placebo response and you do not want to say that out loud.

What actually happened is that your dose fell by half while the number on the box stayed the same. The response is not to stop. It is to raise the dose, which is why carbamazepine is started low and stepped up over the first month or so as a matter of course, and why anyone starting it should be told in advance that the first month is a moving target.

5.2 Where Carbamazepine Came From

It was synthesized in the late 1950s at Geigy in Basel and licensed first for trigeminal neuralgia, a facial pain condition, before its anticonvulsant use was established. Its psychiatric career began in Japan in the 1970s, and its adoption in the West owed a great deal to Robert Post's group at the National Institute of Mental Health, working from the idea that repeated mood episodes might behave something like the kindling of seizures.

That theory has not aged especially well as a complete account. What survived was the observation that carbamazepine did something useful for some patients with bipolar disorder, particularly those who fit the classic picture badly: mixed states, rapid cycling, people with a poor lithium response and no clear family history.

Its place today is honest to state. Ceron-Litvoc and colleagues (2009) reviewed the randomized comparisons against lithium and concluded that carbamazepine was less well supported. Weisler and colleagues (2004) established extended-release carbamazepine as effective in acute mania. It is a genuine second-line drug. It is not a first choice, and if you are on it, you are probably on it because two or three other things were tried first, which is worth knowing because it changes what a switch conversation looks like.

Oxcarbazepine deserves a sentence here, because people confuse the two and prescribers sometimes present the swap as a simple upgrade. Oxcarbazepine is a close chemical relative that induces enzymes less aggressively and does not autoinduce to the same degree. It is easier to live with. It is also less well supported in bipolar disorder than carbamazepine is, which is itself less well supported than lithium. Moving from carbamazepine to oxcarbazepine buys you tolerability and costs you evidence, and that trade should be stated rather than implied.

5.3 What Enzyme Induction Does to the Rest of Your Life

Autoinduction is the small problem. The large one is that carbamazepine does not confine its enzyme induction to itself.

CYP3A4 is not a specialist enzyme. It clears an enormous proportion of everything you will ever swallow. Carbamazepine turning it up means carbamazepine turning down the effective dose of a great many other drugs, silently, without any of them changing.

The one that matters most, and gets missed most, is hormonal contraception.

Carbamazepine is a strong enough inducer to render the combined pill, the progestogen-only pill, the implant, and the patch unreliable (Crawford, 2002; Reimers et al., 2015). Not slightly less effective. Unreliable. Failure rates rise to a degree that means these methods should not be relied on while taking carbamazepine. The methods that are not affected are the ones that do not depend on hepatic metabolism: the copper coil, the hormonal coil, and the injection, with the depot injection requiring closer attention to timing.

Read that against Chapter 4.0 and notice the shape of it. An entire regulatory apparatus was constructed around valproate's reproductive risk. Carbamazepine has a reproductive risk of its own, roughly one percent for neural tube defects (Jentink et al., 2010; Tomson et al., 2018), and it also quietly disables the main method by which people prevent the pregnancies in which that risk would apply. The second of those is the one nobody sends a letter about.

Induction also reduces the effect of some anticoagulants, some antiretrovirals, some immunosuppressants, some antipsychotics, and a long list of other agents. The practical rule is simpler than the list: on carbamazepine, every new prescription and every stopped prescription is an interaction event, and the person best placed to say so at the counter is you.

5.4 Three Other Things Worth Knowing

HLA-B1502. *In 2004, Chung and colleagues reported in Nature that a specific genetic variant, HLA-B*1502, was strongly associated with carbamazepine-induced Stevens-Johnson syndrome in Han Chinese patients. The association turned out to be one of the strongest pharmacogenetic findings in medicine.

Chen and colleagues (2011) then showed that screening for it in Taiwan and avoiding carbamazepine in carriers reduced the incidence of these reactions substantially. The variant is common in some Southeast Asian ancestries and rare in most European ones, which is why testing is recommended based on ancestry rather than universally (Ferrell & McLeod, 2008). If nobody has ever raised this with you and your family origins are in Southeast Asia, it is a fair question to ask.

Hyponatremia. Carbamazepine causes the kidneys to retain water, diluting the sodium in your blood. It is common, it is dose-related, and it is more likely in older people (Van Amelsvoort et al., 1994; Berghuis et al., 2017). The problem is what it looks like: confusion, unsteadiness, a fall, a headache, feeling vague. Nothing about it announces itself as a sodium problem. In an older person it gets attributed to age, or to the illness, or to a different medication, and the fix is a blood test that nobody thought to order.

Blood counts. Carbamazepine carries a small risk of serious blood disorders, which is why full blood counts appear on the monitoring schedule. Tohen and colleagues (1995) put the pharmacoepidemiology of this into proportion across more than 2,000 patients: the severe outcomes are genuinely rare. A mild, stable, non-progressive drop in white cells is common and usually does not require stopping. Sore throat, fever, mouth ulcers, or unexplained bruising do require a blood count today rather than at the next appointment.

There is a fourth thing, and it is the one that connects this chapter to the last one. Carbamazepine and valproate interact in both directions and neither direction is intuitive. Valproate raises the level of carbamazepine's active metabolite while the parent drug's level may look unchanged, so the blood test can be reassuring while the person is getting more drug than the number implies (Bernus et al., 1997). Carbamazepine, meanwhile, induces the enzymes that clear valproate and pulls valproate levels down.

Two drugs, each quietly moving the other, with a laboratory result that does not capture what is happening. This is not a combination to be in without someone who knows the pharmacology paying attention to it.

The following are composite cases.

Case A Garnet started carbamazepine in January. Her psychiatrist spent four minutes explaining that the drug would speed up its own removal, that the dose would rise across the first month, and that the drug appearing to stop working in week four was expected rather than a failure. When it happened, in week four almost exactly, she phoned. The dose went up. She continued.

Case B Rumi started the same drug the same month, from a different service, with no such conversation. In week five her sleep collapsed and her irritability returned. She concluded the drug had failed, which she had half expected, since three previous drugs had failed. She stopped taking it without telling anyone and presented four months later in a mixed state.

The pharmacology was identical in both cases. Both women experienced the same fall in blood level at the same point for the same reason. What differed was four minutes of explanation in January. Rumi did not lack insight or adherence. She interpreted an expected event correctly as a change and incorrectly as a failure, and she had been given nothing that would have let her interpret it otherwise.

5.5 What Happens When the List Gets Long

The following account is a composite, with details changed for anonymity.

Tierney was 61 and had been on carbamazepine for nineteen years. It was, by any reasonable reading, a success. She had a bipolar I diagnosis with a mixed-state history, had failed lithium twice in her thirties, and had been broadly stable since 2007.

What changed was not psychiatric. Over eighteen months she acquired a statin, a blood pressure tablet, and a course of an antibiotic for a dental infection. Each was prescribed sensibly. None was prescribed by anyone who was thinking about carbamazepine.

She presented to her GP with three weeks of feeling vague, one near-fall, and a headache she described as unlike her usual headaches. Her sodium was 124.

The interesting failure here is not that the hyponatremia happened. Carbamazepine and 61 years of age is a well-described combination and the monitoring exists for it. The failure is that the last sodium in her record was from 2019, and that three prescribers in eighteen months had each made a reasonable decision without anyone looking at the whole of her.

Her recovery was uneventful. The dose was reduced, the sodium corrected, and the drug continued, because after nineteen years of stability nobody involved was enthusiastic about finding out what she looked like without it.

What Tierney said afterwards is worth recording, because it names the actual problem. She had assumed that the pharmacy computer was watching for this. Everybody assumes this. The pharmacy computer flags interactions between drugs. It does not flag that a 61-year-old on a long-term inducer has not had her sodium checked in five years, because that is not an interaction, it is an absence, and no system in routine practice is designed to notice an absence.

> **Teaching Point:** *Nineteen years of stability is a reason to protect a drug, not a reason to stop monitoring it.*

> **Teaching Point:** *Hyponatremia on carbamazepine presents as vagueness and falls, not as anything recognizable as an electrolyte problem.*

5.6 The Working Knowledge

Start here: carbamazepine increases the enzymes that clear it, so the dose that worked in week two is delivering roughly half as much by week five, and the drug appearing to fail in the first month is the drug behaving normally rather than the drug failing. That single fact would prevent a great deal of what happened to Rumi.

Build on that: the enzyme it turns up is not private to itself. CYP3A4 clears a large fraction of everything else you take, which makes hormonal contraception unreliable, weakens a long list of other medications, and means that every new prescription in your life is an event that concerns this drug even when nobody in the room is thinking about it.

Then add this: the monitoring that catches the rest of it, sodium, blood counts, liver function, only works if somebody orders it, and after nineteen years of stability nobody orders it, because stability reads to a system as an absence of need. Tierney's sodium was five years old and she was doing well. Those two facts were not in tension. They were the same fact.

The working knowledge for this drug is therefore not pharmacological. It is administrative. You are on a medication whose main risks are produced by things happening elsewhere in your care, by people who are not thinking about it, and the only person present at all of those appointments is you. That is not an ideal design. It is the one you have.

Chapter 6.0 takes the problem one step further out, because most people reading this are not on one of these drugs. They are on two, and nobody has explained the second one either.

Chapter 6.0: Taking More Than One

You are holding four boxes. One of them is a mood stabiliser, and you know what that one is for because somebody told you in 2019. One is an antipsychotic that was added during an admission and never taken away. One is an antidepressant that a GP started at some point, possibly before the bipolar diagnosis existed. The fourth you take at night and you would struggle, under questioning, to say what it does. You have been on some version of this arrangement for six years, it broadly works, and nobody has ever sat down and gone through it with you, because nobody has ever had a reason to.

6.1 How Regimens Actually Get Built

Nobody designs these. That is the first thing to understand, and it explains almost everything about the shape of what you are taking.

The textbook version implies a plan. Assess, select an agent, titrate, review, and if it fails, replace it with the next agent. Clean, sequential, one thing at a time.

What happens instead is accretion. Something gets added during a crisis, when the priority is stopping the crisis and nobody is thinking about 2031. It works, or the crisis ends for reasons nobody can separate from it, and now removing it looks like a risk that nobody has an appetite for. Six months later a different clinician adds something else. The first clinician has moved on. The notes say what was added and rarely say why, and almost never say what would have to be true for it to come off again.

Baldessarini and colleagues (2008) documented the rise of polypharmacy in bipolar disorder over decades, and the drivers are not mysterious. Each individual decision was defensible. The sum of them was never decided by anyone.

The practical consequence is that your regimen has an archaeology rather than a rationale, and the person best placed to excavate it is not your current prescriber, who arrived in year four. It is you, if you have the map. Building that map is the work of this chapter.

6.2 What Each Combination Is Actually Doing

Lithium plus lamotrigine. The commonest maintenance pairing, and the most rational one in this book. Lithium is strongest against the manic pole. Lamotrigine is strongest against the depressive pole. Neither covers both well. Together they cover both, and they do not interact pharmacologically in any meaningful way. Lithium does not change your lamotrigine level and lamotrigine does not change your lithium level. If you are on these two and someone explains the reasoning, it usually lands immediately, because the logic is visible.

Valproate plus lamotrigine. Pharmacologically the opposite situation, as Chapter 3.0 described. Valproate inhibits the enzyme that clears lamotrigine and roughly doubles its concentration. The lamotrigine dose is typically halved and the titration made slower. This combination is used, and it can be the right one, but it requires somebody to have done arithmetic. If your lamotrigine dose did not change when valproate was added, that is a question rather than an oversight to live with.

Lithium plus valproate. The BALANCE trial (2010) tested this directly against each drug alone in bipolar I over two years. The combination outperformed valproate monotherapy. It did not clearly outperform lithium monotherapy. That result is not what most people expect, and it is worth knowing if you are on both: the evidence that the pair beats lithium by itself is weaker than the arrangement implies.

A mood stabiliser plus an antipsychotic. Very common, often reasonable, and frequently a fossil. The antipsychotic went in during an acute episode. Whether it should still be there four years later is a live question that gets asked far less often than it should, and the weight and metabolic cost of the answer is not trivial.

A mood stabiliser plus an antidepressant. The contested one. The ISBD task force reviewed this in detail and reached a position more cautious than routine practice (Pacchiarotti et al., 2013). Sachs and colleagues (2007), in STEP-BD, found adding an antidepressant to a mood stabiliser produced no better outcome than the mood stabiliser alone in bipolar depression. Viktorin and colleagues (2014), using Swedish registry data, found antidepressant monotherapy raised the risk of a switch to mania, while antidepressant plus mood stabiliser did not. The honest summary is that antidepressants in bipolar disorder are not the catastrophe some people claim, are not the help others assume, and should not be taken without a mood stabiliser underneath them.

There is a question underneath all of these that rarely gets asked directly, which is whether more drugs produce more stability. The intuition says yes and the evidence is unimpressed. Post and colleagues (2010) documented just how complex the average regimen required for sustained improvement had become in an outpatient bipolar population, and the finding cuts both ways: some people genuinely need three or four agents, and the field has no reliable way of telling those people apart from the ones who have simply accumulated. Kessing and colleagues (2018), reviewing observational data on maintenance strategies, found lithium monotherapy performing better than several combinations that clinicians reach for first. That does not mean your combination is wrong. It means the assumption that adding is safer than not adding has less behind it than the behavior suggests.

6.3 Drawing the Map

The following worked example uses a composite case.

Calloway, 44, arrived at a medication review taking lithium 800 mg, quetiapine 300 mg at night, sertraline 100 mg, and lamotrigine 100 mg. He had a bipolar I diagnosis dating from 2016.

Step 1: What was known The lithium had been started in 2016 and had a clear rationale. Everything else was less clear.

Step 2: The question that got asked Rather than working from the notes, the clinician drew four boxes on a sheet of paper and asked Calloway to fill in, for each, when it started and what problem it was solving. This is not standard. It takes about ten minutes and it produces information the notes do not contain.

Lithium: 2016, after the second admission. Clear. Quetiapine: 2018, added during a manic relapse, initially 600 mg, reduced to 300 mg at some point Calloway could not date. Purpose then: mania. Purpose now: he took it because it made him sleep. Sertraline: 2015. Started by a GP for what was then thought to be recurrent depression, and never stopped when the diagnosis changed. Nobody had revisited it in nine years. Lamotrigine: 2021, added when the winters kept going badly. Reached 100 mg and stayed there.

Step 3: What the map showed Three things stood out and none of them were in the notes. The sertraline predated the bipolar diagnosis and had never been reviewed against it. The lamotrigine had stopped at 100 mg, which is half the usual maintenance target, for no recorded reason, which meant the drug added for the winters may never have reached a dose that could have helped with the winters. And the quetiapine's current job was sleep, which is a real job, and not the job it was prescribed for.

The complicating moment The obvious move was to stop the sertraline. The clinician did not. Calloway had been on it for nine years, was currently well, and had a low threshold for panic about medication changes. Stopping it would have been defensible and would also have been the fourth thing changing in a regimen that was working. The reasoning offered was: the sertraline is the least defensible drug here and it is also not the one causing you a problem this year.

Step 4: What was done The lamotrigine was raised toward 200 mg, on the grounds that a drug that had never reached a therapeutic dose could not be judged. Nothing else moved. The sertraline question was written down, explicitly, as the next conversation, with a date.

What this worked example shows The map is the intervention. Nothing was deprescribed at that appointment. What changed was that four accumulated decisions became one visible arrangement with a sequence attached, which is more than nine years of notes had produced.

6.4 Where Combinations Break

Three failure patterns account for most of the trouble.

The first is **the unmonitored addition**. A drug goes in and the monitoring for the drug that was already there does not change. Valproate added to lamotrigine without a lamotrigine reduction. A thiazide diuretic added to lithium without a level check for three months. An enzyme inducer added to almost anything. The addition is not the error. The absence of the corresponding adjustment is.

The second is **the orphaned drug**. Something remains in the regimen because removing it requires a decision and continuing it does not. Every prescriber in the chain inherits it, none of them started it, and none of them wants to be the one who stopped it three weeks before a relapse. This is a system producing a predictable outcome from rational individual behavior, and the fact that it is nobody's fault does not make it less of a problem for the person swallowing four tablets.

The third is **attribution collapse**. On four psychotropics, you cannot tell which one is causing what. The tremor could be lithium or it could be the sertraline. The weight could be quetiapine, could be lithium, could be an undiagnosed thyroid problem, could be the depression. The sedation could be any of them. When something goes wrong on a complex regimen, the diagnostic power of the situation is very close to zero, and it does not recover until something is simplified.

Attribution collapse is the one that costs the most and gets discussed the least. It has a corollary worth stating: the more drugs you are on, the less your prescriber can learn from anything that happens to you. A regimen of four is not four times as informative as a regimen of one. It is considerably less informative, because every outcome has four candidate explanations and no way to test between them. Simplification is not only about side effects. It is about restoring the ability of your treatment to tell you anything.

6.5 Simplifying Without Blowing It Up

The following account is a composite, with details changed for anonymity.

Oakley had been well for five years on lithium and olanzapine. He was also 40 pounds heavier than he had been in 2019, prediabetic, and had reached the point of saying that he would rather be unwell than continue as he was, which is a sentence prescribers should take literally rather than as a figure of speech.

The plan was to withdraw the olanzapine slowly over six months while the lithium continued.

It went wrong at month four. Not dramatically. His sleep fragmented, he became irritable, and his wife noticed before he did, which is a pattern Chapter 13.0 has a good deal more to say about.

What happened next is the part worth attending to. The taper was not abandoned. It was paused at the dose he had reached, held for eight weeks until things settled, and then resumed at a slower rate. The total time was fourteen months rather than six. He came off it.

The temptation at month four was to conclude that the olanzapine was necessary and restore the original dose. That reading was available and it was probably wrong. What the wobble showed was that the rate was too fast, which is a different finding from the drug being required, and telling those two apart is most of the skill in deprescribing.

Oakley lost 22 pounds over the following year. His prediabetes did not fully reverse. He is on lithium alone and has not relapsed, and he is entirely aware that this could change, and he considers the trade worth it. That last part is his judgment to make, and it is worth noticing that nobody could have made it for him.

> **Teaching Point:** *A wobble during a taper is information about the rate, not proof of necessity.*
>
> **Teaching Point:** *"I would rather be unwell than continue like this" is a clinical statement. It means the current arrangement has already failed on a dimension nobody is measuring.*

6.6 Bringing It Together

The practical upshot is a single piece of homework and one rule.

The homework is the map. Four boxes, or however many you have. For each: what it is, when it started, what problem it was solving, and who added it. Do it on paper before your next appointment rather than in the appointment, because ten minutes of your time is available and ten minutes of theirs is not. You will find at least one drug you cannot account for. Almost everyone does. That drug is your next conversation.

The rule is: one change at a time, and long enough to know. Complex regimens hide their own effects, and the only way to learn anything from a change is to make one change and then wait longer than feels comfortable. Two simultaneous changes produce an outcome that teaches you nothing about either.

And a caution that belongs to this chapter rather than any of the drug chapters. Nothing in here is a reason to stop something yourself. Calloway's sertraline was the least defensible drug in his regimen and it was also not the thing to touch that year. Oakley's taper needed fourteen months and a clinician holding the rate. Both of those are judgments made with someone, not despite them.

Chapter 7.0 goes after the one category of interaction that will not wait for an appointment, because it happens in a supermarket, on a holiday, or on the fourth day of a stomach bug.

Chapter 7.0: Ibuprofen and Other Ordinary Risks

The apartment had air conditioning but Dune had not worked out how to make it come on, and by the fourth day it did not seem worth the trouble of asking. It was 34 degrees outside and had been all week. She had burned her shoulders on day two, badly enough that sleeping was uncomfortable, and had bought a box of ibuprofen from a pharmacy near the beach, where the assistant spoke enough English to point at the shelf. She had taken two, three times a day, for three days. She was drinking, but mostly in the evenings, and mostly wine. On the morning of the fifth day her hands would not do what she asked them to, and she vomited twice before ten o'clock, and she thought, with total sincerity, that she had food poisoning.

7.1 What Dune Did

Nothing on that list looks like a medical decision.

She went on holiday. She got sunburned. She bought a painkiller from a pharmacy shelf, which is what the shelf is for. She had some wine. She did not drink as much water as she would have at home, because at home she was not at the beach and did not have to think about it. And she kept taking her lithium, at the same dose, at the same time, because she had been taking it at the same dose at the same time for four years and it had never caused her a problem.

Every one of those was reasonable in isolation. Together they raised her lithium level far enough to make her toxic.

She was in a hospital in a country whose language she did not speak, explaining through a translation app that she took a medicine for her mood, and it took eleven hours before anyone measured the thing that was actually wrong with her. Her level was 2.1 mmol/L.

7.2 The Four Things That Happened

Take them apart, because each one is a mechanism and each one is available to you at home.

The heat. Sweating loses water and sodium. Chapter 2.0 made the point that your kidneys handle lithium as though it were sodium; when your body decides sodium is scarce, it holds on to sodium harder, and it holds on to lithium at the same time, because it cannot tell the difference. Hot weather is a lithium-raising event. So is a fever. So is a sauna, a long run, or a physically hard day on a building site in August.

The reduced fluid. The same mechanism, arriving from the other direction.

The ibuprofen. This is the big one and it is the one nobody is warned about. Nonsteroidal anti-inflammatory drugs reduce lithium clearance by the kidney, and the effect is not trivial. Ragheb (1990) documented the clinical significance of this interaction, and Finley (2016), reviewing lithium interactions comprehensively, places NSAIDs among the most important. Ibuprofen, naproxen, diclofenac, and the rest can raise a lithium level substantially over days. They are sold on open shelves in every country Dune has ever visited.

The alcohol. A modest contributor here, mostly through dehydration rather than any direct pharmacological effect, and it earns its place on the list because it makes everything else on the list worse rather than because it is dangerous by itself.

Four ordinary things. Compounding. None of them requiring a prescription, a decision, or a moment where a reasonable person would have thought to check.

7.3 The Concept Is a Narrow Window

Chapter 2.0 introduced the **narrow therapeutic index**, and Dune's holiday is what that phrase means when it stops being a phrase.

Most drugs have a wide margin. You can be moderately dehydrated on ramipril and nothing happens. You can take ibuprofen alongside most antidepressants indefinitely. The system tolerates disturbance because there is room in it.

Lithium has no room. The distance between a working level and a dangerous one is a factor of about two and a half, and the variables that move you across that distance are not medical events. They are weather, illness, exercise, diet, and the contents of a pharmacy shelf. Juurlink and colleagues (2004), in a population-based study of drug-induced lithium toxicity in older adults, found that the culprits were mostly ordinary prescriptions issued for ordinary reasons: diuretics, ACE inhibitors, and NSAIDs.

That is the concept this chapter is built on and it is worth stating plainly because it inverts the usual advice. The danger is not that you will do something dramatic. The danger is that you will do something completely unremarkable, several times, in a week when the weather is bad for you.

7.4 The List Worth Knowing

NSAIDs. Ibuprofen, naproxen, diclofenac, and the topical versions in smaller measure. Raise lithium. Paracetamol, called acetaminophen in the United States, does not, and is the safer first reach for ordinary pain.

ACE inhibitors and ARBs. The blood pressure drugs ending in "-pril" and "-sartan." Raise lithium, sometimes considerably, and sometimes weeks after starting (Handler, 2009). This is what happened to Arden in Chapter 2.0.

Thiazide diuretics. Bendroflumethiazide, hydrochlorothiazide. These raise lithium levels typically by 50 to 100 percent. That is not a nudge. That is a dose doubling arriving through a blood pressure prescription. They are not forbidden, and Chapter 11.0 discusses why one particular diuretic is sometimes deliberately added, but a thiazide plus lithium requires a level check within a fortnight rather than at the next review.

Dehydration in all its forms. Gastroenteritis. Fever. Heat. Hard exercise. Alcohol. Any of these lasting more than a day is a reason to think about your level rather than a reason to feel unwell in peace.

Sudden dietary sodium change. Starting a low-salt diet raises your lithium level. So does a crash diet. So, occasionally, does a sudden change in the other direction. Your kidney set the lithium equilibrium against your usual salt intake. Change the salt and you have changed the drug.

Alcohol, honestly. There is no direct interaction of significance. Lithium and alcohol do not fight each other in your bloodstream. What alcohol does is dehydrate you, disturb your sleep, and destabilize your mood, and the third of those is the one that matters most for someone with bipolar disorder. That is a real argument. It is a different argument from the one people expect, and pretending there is a pharmacological catastrophe where there is not tends to cost the clinician credibility for the argument that is actually true.

If you are not on lithium. Most of this chapter is a lithium chapter, because lithium is the drug in this book with the narrow window and the kidney handling that makes ordinary life dangerous. The other three have their own everyday list and it is shorter.

For valproate, the ordinary risk is alcohol, and the reason is the liver rather than the level. Valproate is metabolized hepatically and carries a small risk of liver injury; sustained heavy drinking on valproate is a genuinely poor combination in a way that a glass of wine is not. Aspirin, of all things, displaces valproate from its binding proteins and raises the free fraction, which is a fact almost nobody knows and which matters most in older people taking low-dose aspirin daily.

For carbamazepine, the ordinary risk is grapefruit juice, which sounds like folklore and is not. Grapefruit inhibits the enzyme carbamazepine depends on and can raise its level meaningfully. The larger ordinary risk, as Chapter 5.0 set out, is any new prescription at all.

For lamotrigine, the everyday list is close to empty, which is one of its quiet virtues. Hormonal contraception is the exception worth knowing: the combined pill lowers lamotrigine levels by roughly half, and the pill-free week raises them again, which means a woman on both can be riding a monthly wave in her lamotrigine level that nobody has mentioned to her. Starting or stopping the pill on lamotrigine is a dose event.

7.5 What Should Have Been Different

The following is a composite case; identifying details have been changed.

Background Umber, 52, on lithium for nine years, level historically stable around 0.7 mmol/L. No prior toxicity.

Presentation He attended his GP with three days of vomiting and diarrhea, presumed viral. He was mildly unsteady on his feet, which he and the GP both attributed to the illness. He was advised to take fluids and rest. No blood was taken.

Analysis Both of them made the same error, which is that they treated the gastroenteritis as the problem. For a person on lithium, three days of vomiting is not primarily an infection. It is a lithium event, in which the infection is the mechanism. The unsteadiness was the finding that should have moved things, because ataxia in a lithium patient during dehydration is not a symptom of gastroenteritis, it is the first line of the toxicity list.

Intervention He returned two days later, worse. A level was finally taken and came back at 1.6 mmol/L. He was admitted for fluids and his lithium was held for four days. He did not require dialysis. He recovered fully.

Outcome The lithium was restarted at his previous dose and his level returned to baseline within a fortnight. What did not return to baseline was his confidence, and he spent the following year checking himself for symptoms in a way he had never done before, which is its own kind of cost and does not appear in any outcome measure.

> **Teaching Point:** *Any illness causing fluid loss in a lithium patient is a lithium problem wearing the clothes of the presenting complaint.*
>
> **Teaching Point:** *Unsteadiness during dehydration on lithium is not attributable to the dehydration until a level says so.*
>
> **Teaching Point:** *A near-miss produces a lasting anxiety that nobody schedules a follow-up for.*

There is one more everyday category, and it is the one people find hardest to hear. Surgery, imaging, and dental work all involve clinicians who will not think about your mood stabiliser because it is not what they are there for. An anesthetist needs to know about lithium. A radiologist giving you contrast needs to know about your kidney function. A surgeon starving you of fluids from midnight needs to know that you are taking a drug whose level rises when you are dry. None of them will ask in a way that gets the answer, for the same reason Arden's ramipril went unmentioned in Chapter 2.0: the question people ask is about medicines, and patients hear medicines as meaning the ones relevant to the person asking.

7.6 The Sick Day Rule

Write this down now, while you are well, and put it somewhere it will be found by someone who is not well.

If you cannot keep fluids down, or you have had diarrhea, fever, or heavy sweating for more than about 24 hours: contact your prescriber or an out-of-hours service, tell them you take lithium before you tell them anything else, and ask for a level. If you cannot reach anyone and you are becoming unsteady, drowsy, or your tremor has changed character, that is an emergency department, today, and you say the word lithium in the first sentence.

If you are unwell but managing, keep taking fluids with some salt in them rather than plain water alone, and do not decide by yourself to skip doses. Skipping is sometimes right and it is a decision that needs someone with your level in front of them.

And a script for the pharmacy counter, which is the single highest-yield sentence in this book. Every time, in every country, before anything is handed over: **I take lithium. Is this safe with lithium?** Not "I take medication for my mental health," which will get you a sympathetic nod and a box of ibuprofen. The word lithium. Pharmacists know exactly what it means and their software will do the rest.

7.7 Closing the Loop

Dune got the air conditioning working eventually, because a nurse in the hospital wrote the instructions down on a piece of paper for her, which was the single most useful medical intervention of the entire holiday.

What she says now about that week is not that she made a mistake. She is quite firm about this, and I think she is right. There was no mistake. There was a woman on holiday who got sunburned and bought some painkillers, and every individual thing she did was the thing a reasonable person does. The failure was not hers. It was that in four years of lithium treatment, across probably thirty appointments, nobody had ever said the word ibuprofen to her.

That is a fixable problem and it costs about forty seconds. It did not happen for Dune, it did not happen for Umber, and the reason is not negligence. It is that this conversation belongs to nobody in particular: too practical for the psychiatrist, too psychiatric for the GP, and invisible to the pharmacist because the box came off a shelf and no prescription was ever written.

So it falls to you, which is unfair and is also the situation. Six words at every pharmacy counter. A sick day plan written while well. A note in your wallet. That is the whole of the defense, and it would have been enough on day two in that apartment, before the shoulders, before the box, before the fifth morning.

Chapter 8.0 stays in the same territory but changes the question. Dune's level was 2.1 before anyone thought to measure it. Somebody should have known what they were looking at, and the person best placed to know was not a clinician.

Chapter 8.0: Knowing Toxicity When You See It

A woman whose husband has bipolar disorder once described the moment she understood something was wrong. It was not the vomiting, she said, and it was not that he seemed confused, because he had seemed confused before and it had meant nothing. It was that his hands were doing something different. He had always had a slight tremor, for years, and she had stopped seeing it the way you stop seeing a picture on your own wall. This was not that. This was bigger and slower and it came in bursts, and she could not have told a doctor why it frightened her. She just knew that the wrong thing was happening, and she was ten hours ahead of anyone else who saw him.

8.1 Two Different Emergencies

Lithium toxicity is not one event. It comes in two shapes, and telling them apart matters, because they behave differently and they arrive by different routes.

Acute toxicity is an overdose. Somebody takes a large quantity at once, deliberately or otherwise. The stomach and gut symptoms come first and dominate: vomiting, diarrhea, abdominal pain. The neurological picture arrives later, because the lithium has to leave the blood and get into brain tissue, and that takes hours.

Chronic toxicity is what happened to Dune in Chapter 7.0 and to Umber. The dose has not changed. Something else has: the weather, an illness, a new tablet, a dry week. The level creeps up over days while the tissue concentration climbs alongside it. There is often little vomiting. The neurology comes first and it comes quietly.

Chronic toxicity is more dangerous at a lower number, which is the single most counterintuitive fact in this chapter. A person who has swallowed a bottle can survive a level of 3.0 in reasonable shape, because the lithium has not had time to reach the brain. A person on maintenance who has drifted to 1.8 over eight days can be considerably more unwell, because their brain has been marinating. Ott and colleagues (2016), following lithium intoxication in a population cohort, found the clinical course tracked the pattern more than the number.

That is why "what is your level" is the second question and not the first. The first question is how long.

8.2 The Signs in the Order They Come

Early. The tremor changes. This is the finding that matters most and it is the one nobody explains. A fine, fast, low-amplitude tremor is a normal, common side effect of lithium; something like a third of people have one, it is present at rest, and it is not a warning. What is a warning is when that tremor changes character: becomes coarse, larger, slower, more like a shake than a buzz. Alongside it: nausea, loose stools, a general feeling of being unwell without a location.

Middle. Unsteadiness. Ataxia, which means walking as though drunk, veering, misjudging the doorframe. Slurred speech. Drowsiness that is not tiredness. Muscle twitching. This is the point at which a bystander notices, and it is the point at which the person themselves usually does not, because the same lithium that is affecting their gait is affecting their judgment about their gait.

Late. Confusion. Marked disorientation. Seizures. Reduced consciousness. Kidney failure. This is an intensive care presentation and the interval from the middle stage to here can be short.

There is a rare late outcome worth naming, because people find out about it by accident and it terrifies them more in ignorance. A small number of people who have had severe lithium neurotoxicity are left with permanent problems, chiefly with coordination, and there is a literature on it under the acronym SILENT (Adityanjee et al., 2005). It is rare. It is also one of the strongest arguments in this book for acting at the middle stage rather than the late one, because the difference between full recovery and not is usually hours.

8.3 The Distinction That Prevents Panic

"My level is 1.1" and "I am toxic" are different statements. People conflate them and then spend a weekend frightened for no reason.

A level slightly above the maintenance range in a person who feels fine is a dose question. It gets a repeat test, a look at what changed, and probably a small adjustment. It is not an emergency and it does not mean damage has occurred.

Toxicity is a clinical state. It is defined by how the person is, not by the number, and this cuts both ways: people have been toxic at 1.3 and people have been fine at 1.6. The number contributes to the picture. It does not constitute it.

The practical version: if the number is high and you feel completely normal, phone in the morning. If you feel wrong, in the ways described in 8.2, the number is irrelevant to what you should do next, including if the number is unknown, including if the last number was fine.

There is a second distinction that saves people from a different kind of unnecessary fear. A single episode of chronic toxicity, caught at the middle stage and treated, does not commit you to kidney disease. Kirkham and colleagues (2014) found that a level above 1.0 mmol/L was followed by an acute drop in eGFR, which sounds alarming and is worth taking seriously, and Chapter 9.0

puts it in the context of what happens over decades rather than over one bad fortnight. Ott and colleagues (2016), following renal function after intoxication episodes, found the picture less catastrophic than the folklore. What the folklore gets right is that repeated episodes accumulate. What it gets wrong is that one is a life sentence.

8.4 What to Do, in Order

The following worked example uses a composite case.

Zephyr, 58, had been on lithium for twelve years. His daughter phoned him on a Sunday and thought he sounded drunk. He had not been drinking.

Step 1: What she noticed Slurred speech on the phone. That was all. No other information.

Step 2: What she did that was right She drove over rather than reasoning about it. Twenty minutes. When she arrived he was unsteady getting out of the chair and his hands were shaking coarsely, and he told her he was fine and had a bit of a bug.

Step 3: The moment it could have gone wrong He refused to go anywhere. He was not being difficult; he genuinely believed he was fine, which is exactly what lithium does to your assessment of whether you are fine. His daughter had two options: negotiate, or override.

The complicating moment She overrode him. She has since said that the only reason she felt able to do that was a conversation eighteen months earlier, at a kitchen table, when he was well, in which he had said out loud that if she ever thought he was toxic she should ignore whatever he said at the time. He had thought it a slightly theatrical thing to be asked to say. It turned out to be the entire mechanism.

Step 4: What she said on the phone This part matters and it is teachable. She did not say "my father is confused" or "my father is unwell." She said: **he takes lithium, he is unsteady and slurring, he has had diarrhea for two days, I think he is toxic.** Four facts, in eleven seconds. The word lithium in the first clause.

Step 5: What happened Level 1.9. Fluids, lithium held for three days, no dialysis. Home in four days.

What this worked example shows The clinical skill in this episode belonged entirely to a woman with no medical training. What she had was a list of signs, a sentence to say on the phone, and permission granted in advance. All three were free. All three were obtained at a kitchen table on a day when nothing was wrong.

8.5 Where the Recognition Fails

The following account is a composite, with details changed for anonymity.

Nyx was 71 and lived alone. She had been on lithium for thirty years and on a blood pressure tablet for six. In February she had a chest infection, was prescribed antibiotics, ate very little for a week, and was found by a neighbor on the floor of her hallway.

The difficulty in her case was not that the signs were absent. They were all there: she had been unsteady for four days, and two different people had seen her be unsteady. The difficulty is that she was 71, and every sign of lithium toxicity in an older person has a more available explanation. Unsteadiness is age. Confusion is a urinary infection or the beginning of dementia. Drowsiness is the chest infection. Tremor is old.

Juurlink and colleagues (2004) documented this population specifically, and the picture is consistent: older adults on lithium become toxic through ordinary prescriptions and ordinary illnesses, and the presentation is systematically misattributed because everything it looks like is also something that happens to people of that age.

Nyx recovered, slowly, and did not return to living alone. Whether the toxicity caused that or accelerated something already moving is not answerable, and her family have had to live with the not knowing, which in my experience is harder than most clinicians appreciate.

> **Teaching Point:** *In an older person, every sign of lithium toxicity has a competing explanation that is more common and less dangerous. That is precisely why the level must be measured rather than reasoned about.*
>
> **Teaching Point:** *Living alone is a clinical risk factor for lithium toxicity, and it appears on no monitoring form anywhere.*

8.6 The Emergencies on the Other Three

Toxicity is a lithium word. The other three drugs have their own emergency lists, shorter and sharper, and they belong here rather than buried in their own chapters.

Lamotrigine. Rash with fever, mucosal involvement, or systemic illness, in the first two months. Chapter 3.0 set this out in full. Stop and be seen today.

Valproate. Two things. Persistent vomiting with abdominal pain radiating to the back can be pancreatitis, which is rare and serious. Jaundice, dark urine, unusual bruising, or profound lethargy can be liver injury, which is rare, more common in the first six months, and more common in children than adults. Neither presents in a way that announces which drug is responsible, and both are worth naming out loud to whoever is assessing you.

Carbamazepine. Also two. Fever with a sore throat or mouth ulcers, which needs a full blood count today rather than a course of antibiotics. And the hyponatremia described in Chapter 5.0, which presents as confusion, unsteadiness, or a fall, and which will be attributed to almost anything before someone checks a sodium.

The pattern across all four is identical and worth extracting. In every case, the emergency presents as something extremely ordinary: a rash, a sore throat, a stomach upset, a fall. In every case, the ordinary explanation is more likely than the drug. And in every case, the thing that distinguishes them is a test that takes ten minutes and will not be ordered unless somebody names the drug.

8.7 The Takeaways That Matter

Four things, and then this chapter is done.

Learn your own tremor. Look at your hands now, while everything is fine. That baseline is a piece of clinical information and you are the only person who has it. A change in the character of that tremor, coarser and slower, is the earliest usable sign there is.

Grant permission in advance. The conversation Zephyr had at his kitchen table was worth more than every monitoring appointment he attended that decade. Say the sentence out loud to somebody: if you think I am toxic, act, and ignore what I tell you at the time. It sounds melodramatic on the day you say it. It is not melodramatic. It is the only thing that works, because the drug takes away the judgment you would need to consent at the moment consent is required.

Learn the phone sentence. Lithium, then the signs, then the duration. Not "my mood medication." Not "he seems off." The word first, because it changes what happens at the other end of the line within seconds.

Do not wait for the number. Every case in this chapter and the last one contains an interval in which somebody sensible waited for information before acting. Dune waited for the vomiting to stop. Umber and his GP waited for the virus to pass. Nyx's neighbors waited to see if she would be better tomorrow. The waiting was the injury. If someone on lithium is unsteady and slurring, the level can be measured after they are in the building.

Chapter 9.0 turns from the emergency to the slow question, and to the one number in this book that people carry around for a decade without ever being told what it means.

Chapter 9.0: The Kidney Conversation

Long-term lithium treatment causes progressive kidney damage in a small number of people, and the risk rises the longer you take it. Long-term lithium treatment has not been shown to reduce kidney function meaningfully compared with the alternatives, and the association may owe more to bipolar disorder itself than to the drug. Both of those statements come from good research groups. Both have been published in serious journals in the last decade. Neither is fringe. If you have spent an evening searching for an answer to this question and come away more confused than you started, that is not a failure of your search. You found the actual state of the evidence.

9.1 The Question That Is Actually Being Asked

Start by separating two things that get conflated in every conversation about this, including most clinical ones.

Nephrogenic diabetes insipidus is common. Lithium interferes with the kidney's ability to concentrate urine in response to the hormone that tells it to. The result is that you produce large volumes of dilute urine and are thirsty all the time. Somewhere between 20 and 40 percent of people on long-term lithium have some degree of this. It is unpleasant, it is inconvenient, it wakes you up at night, and it is largely reversible on stopping. It is not kidney damage in the sense people mean when they are frightened.

Chronic tubulointerstitial nephropathy is the other thing. Slow scarring of kidney tissue over years, showing up as a declining eGFR, and progressing in a small proportion of people to end-stage renal failure and dialysis. Markowitz and colleagues (2000) characterized the histology directly in biopsy specimens, and it is a real, describable entity.

They are different. They are not stages of the same process, they do not have the same prognosis, and one of them is a nuisance while the other is a threat. When a clinician says "lithium can affect the kidneys," they are usually saying something true about both and useful about neither, and the patient goes home having heard the second one.

The debate is about the second one.

9.2 The Case That the Risk Is Real

Bendz and colleagues (2010) put the question fairly in the title of their paper: renal failure occurs in chronic lithium treatment but is uncommon. That is the position at its most honest. It happens. Not often.

The evidence for it is duration. Golic and colleagues (2023), following a lithium-treated population from a Swedish hospital laboratory database, found the relationship with time to be steep. Twenty or more years of lithium exposure carried an odds ratio of 6.14 for severe kidney disease compared with one to five years of exposure, with a confidence interval running from 2.65 to 14.26. That is not a subtle finding.

They also found something else useful: pre-treatment creatinine predicted risk. People whose creatinine sat in the upper third of the normal reference range before they ever took lithium had a hazard ratio of 4.6 compared with those in the lower third. In other words, some of this is about the kidney you started with.

Presne and colleagues (2003) described the rate of progression and its prognostic factors, and the picture that emerges from that literature is of a slow process, over decades, in a minority, with a strong relationship to cumulative exposure and to episodes of toxicity. Schoretsanitis and colleagues (2022), pooling the literature in a systematic review, found the prevalence of impaired kidney function in long-term lithium patients considerably higher than the general population rate.

The strongest version of this position is not "lithium destroys kidneys." It is: this is a slow, duration-dependent process affecting a minority, it is measurable years before it matters, and the people who dismiss it are usually looking at cohorts followed for ten years when the relevant timescale is thirty.

9.3 The Case That the Risk Is Overstated

Kessing and colleagues (2015), using nationwide Danish registry data, examined the rate of chronic kidney disease in people using lithium and in people using anticonvulsants. If lithium were the driver, lithium users should stand out. They did not stand out in the way the hypothesis predicts. The finding pointed toward something about the population rather than something about the drug.

That is the crux of this position and it is a serious argument. Bipolar disorder is independently associated with kidney disease. People with bipolar disorder have higher rates of hypertension, diabetes, obesity, and smoking, all of which are far better established causes of chronic kidney disease than any psychiatric medication. Parsaik and colleagues (2025), following 1,603 patients on long-term lithium, found that 15.3 percent developed chronic kidney disease of stage three or worse, and that the significant risk factors were hypertension, age, and having bipolar disorder. Notice what is doing the work in that list.

Clos and colleagues (2015), in a population-based cohort study published in The Lancet Psychiatry, examined the long-term effect of lithium maintenance on eGFR and did not find the deterioration the older literature predicted. Aiff and colleagues (2014) went further and argued that modern treatment principles, meaning lower target levels, once-daily dosing, and actual monitoring, may have eliminated lithium-induced renal failure as a meaningful problem. Their later work (2015, and the 2023 analysis of early renal damage across three decades of cohorts) found low rates that had not changed over time even as monitoring improved.

The strongest version of this position: the frightening figures come from patients treated in the 1960s and 1970s at levels nobody would use now, with monitoring nobody would accept now, and applying them to a person started on lithium in 2015 at a target of 0.7 mmol/L is a category error.

9.4 Where the Evidence Actually Runs Out

Three things are true simultaneously and the field has not reconciled them.

The duration signal is real and it is large. Six-fold at twenty years is not noise, and the studies that fail to find lithium effects are frequently too short to see it. Ten years of follow-up on a process that takes twenty-five is not evidence of absence.

The confounding is also real and it is severe. Bipolar disorder brings hypertension and metabolic disease with it, and lithium is preferentially given to people who stay in treatment for decades, who are therefore older and sicker by the time anyone counts. Untangling drug from disorder from duration in observational data is not a problem that better statistics will solve. It would require a randomized trial running thirty years, which will not happen.

And the absolute numbers are small. This is the part that gets lost in the argument. Golic and colleagues found that for people starting lithium between 18 and 54, the ten-year cumulative risk of severe kidney disease ranged from zero to 0.7 percent. Zero to seven in a thousand, over a decade. The lifetime risk figures rise substantially for people starting lithium in later life, reaching 13.9 to 18.6 percent for those starting between 55 and 74, which is a genuinely different conversation and one that older patients are rarely given.

Werneke and colleagues (2012) did the most useful thing anyone has done with this question, which was to stop arguing about it and run a decision analysis. They modeled the risk of renal failure against the risk of relapse and suicide from stopping. The conclusion was not close. For most patients, continuing lithium came out ahead, because the thing on the other side of the ledger is not "nothing," it is a disorder that kills people.

Then Parsaik and colleagues (2025) added the finding that should reframe the entire discussion, and which almost nobody has absorbed. In their cohort, among patients who developed chronic kidney disease, stopping lithium did not change the subsequent course of their kidney function.

Sit with that. If it holds, the conversation "should I stop lithium to protect my kidneys" may be built on a premise that does not survive contact with the data. You would be giving up the drug and keeping the kidney disease.

Except that it may not hold, and the counter-evidence arrived almost immediately. Fransson and colleagues (2025), using a mirror-image design on the Swedish LiSIE cohort and looking at patients who stopped lithium and in some cases restarted it, found that stopping slowed the rate of eGFR decline. That is the opposite of Parsaik's finding, published within months of it, from a group that includes the same authors who produced the decision analysis discussed above. Two good studies, two directions, one year.

What that means practically is that the single question a patient most wants answered, will stopping help my kidney, currently has two credible answers and no way to choose between them from the outside. Fransson's own conclusion is the most honest sentence in this literature: what is needed is a patient-centred rather than a kidney-centred approach, because the potential for an improved kidney prognosis has to be weighed against a worse psychiatric course, relapse, and suicide.

9.5 What This Looks Like in a Room

The following is a composite case; identifying details have been changed.

Background Wren, 49, bipolar I, on lithium for seventeen years with no episodes since year two. Two prior admissions before lithium, one following a serious suicide attempt at 30.

Presentation Routine bloods showed eGFR 57, down from 78 six years earlier. Her GP wrote to her psychiatrist recommending that lithium be stopped. Wren received a copy of the letter before either clinician had spoken to her about it, which is how a large number of people find out about this.

Analysis Her eGFR trend was real and it was going in one direction. She had also been hypertensive for nine years and had gained 30 pounds over the same period. Attributing the decline to lithium alone was not supportable. Attributing none of it to lithium was not supportable either.

Against that sat a history containing a near-fatal attempt, and the antisuicidal evidence reviewed in Chapter 1.0.

Intervention Three things were done and one was refused. Her blood pressure was treated properly for the first time, which had a larger evidence base for protecting her kidney than stopping lithium did. Her lithium dose was reduced, with a target at the lower end of the range, since dose and cumulative exposure carry the signal. She was referred to a nephrologist, jointly rather than as a handover. And the request to stop was declined, with the reasoning written down and given to her.

Outcome At two years her eGFR was 55. Essentially flat. She remains on lithium. She has not relapsed. Nobody can say whether this was the right call, and that uncertainty is permanent.

> **Teaching Point:** *The first intervention for a falling eGFR in a lithium patient is often the blood pressure, not the lithium.*
>
> **Teaching Point:** *A nephrology referral is not a decision to stop. It is the acquisition of someone who knows more about kidneys than anyone else in the conversation.*
>
> **Teaching Point:** *"Stop the lithium" arriving as a letter rather than a conversation is a failure of process that patients experience as a verdict.*

The following account is a composite, with details changed for anonymity.

Ellis had the same numbers as Wren, more or less, and made the opposite choice.

He was 44, his eGFR had gone from 82 to 59 over eight years, and he had a bipolar II diagnosis. No admissions. No suicide attempts. Two depressive episodes in twelve years, both managed as an outpatient. He had also spent those twelve years thirsty, urinating six or seven times a night, and hating it in a way he had never quite managed to convey in a ten-minute appointment.

He came off lithium over nine months. He went onto lamotrigine. His eGFR stopped falling and settled at 61, where it has stayed. He has had one depressive episode since, in year two, which was significant and did not require admission.

The point of putting Ellis next to Wren is not that one of them was right. It is that the numbers were almost identical and the decisions were both correct, because the numbers were never the input that mattered. Wren had a near-fatal attempt in her history and Ellis did not. That single fact, which appears nowhere in a renal function panel, is what the decision actually turned on.

> **Teaching Point:** *Identical laboratory data supports opposite decisions, and the difference lives in the psychiatric history rather than the renal one.*
>
> **Teaching Point:** *The nephrogenic diabetes insipidus that nobody counts as damage was, for Ellis, the largest single cost of the drug.*

9.6 Where This Leaves Us

Settled, or close enough to act on:

Nephrogenic diabetes insipidus is common, unpleasant, and largely reversible. Progressive nephropathy is uncommon. Risk rises with duration and with cumulative exposure, and episodes of toxicity contribute. Pre-treatment kidney function predicts who is vulnerable. Starting lithium after 55 carries a different, higher risk profile than starting at 25, and older patients are rarely told this. And the trend across years is the clinical object; a single eGFR is close to meaningless.

Contested, and honestly so:

Whether lithium adds risk beyond what bipolar disorder, hypertension, and age contribute on their own. Kessing's registry data and Clos's cohort say the addition is small or absent; Golic's duration data says otherwise; both are looking at real patients and neither can randomize.

Whether the old figures apply to modern treatment. Aiff's group argues the risk has been engineered out by lower targets and better monitoring, and the argument is decent, and it is also exactly what you would expect a group to conclude from cohorts that are not yet old enough.

And the largest open question, which is whether stopping helps at all once the damage is established. Parsaik (2025) suggests it may not. Fransson (2025) suggests it may. Those two papers are months apart and point opposite ways, which means that anyone who tells you confidently that stopping will protect your kidney, or confidently that it will not, is ahead of the evidence in one direction or the other.

What you can do with this is narrower than it looks. Plot your own eGFR over time, because nobody else will. Get your blood pressure treated, because it is doing more damage than the lithium is and it is easier to fix. Ask what your creatinine was before you started, because it predicts your risk and it is sitting in a file. And if someone proposes stopping to protect your kidney, ask the question the evidence now supports asking: what do you expect my kidney to do differently if I stop?

They may not have an answer. That is not a reason to disregard them. It is a reason to have the conversation properly, with a nephrologist in it, rather than by letter.

Chapter 10.0 goes after the other organ on the monitoring form, the one that produces symptoms everybody blames on the illness for years at a time.

Chapter 10.0: Thyroid Calcium and Tiredness

How would you tell the difference between a depressive episode and an underactive thyroid, from the inside? Not in a textbook. In your own body, on a Tuesday in November, when you have been tired for four months, gained eleven pounds without changing anything, cannot get warm, cannot concentrate, and have stopped answering messages. Both conditions produce exactly that. The question is not rhetorical and it is not academic: on lithium, both are considerably more likely than they would otherwise be, one of them is a two-minute fix, and the other one is going to get you a change to your psychiatric medication that will not help. Nothing you can feel distinguishes them. Nothing your psychiatrist can observe distinguishes them either.

10.1 What Lithium Does to the Thyroid

Your thyroid makes hormone. To release it, the gland needs to do something that lithium interferes with directly. Lithium concentrates in thyroid tissue and blocks the release of thyroid hormone into the bloodstream. Your pituitary notices the shortfall and responds by producing more **thyroid stimulating hormone**, or TSH, which is a signal telling the thyroid to work harder.

That is why TSH is the number on your form rather than the thyroid hormone itself. TSH is the shouting. A rising TSH means the pituitary is raising its voice at a gland that is not responding properly, and it rises before the hormone levels fall far enough to be obviously abnormal. It is an early warning system, which is exactly what you want on a six-monthly blood test.

The frequency is not trivial. Estimates vary with how you define the outcome, but somewhere in the region of 6 to 20 percent of people on long-term lithium develop clinical hypothyroidism, and considerably more develop subclinical changes or thyroid antibodies (Kirov et al., 2005; Johnston & Eagles, 1999). Shine and colleagues (2015), examining laboratory data from nearly 5,000 lithium-treated patients, found the association with thyroid dysfunction clearly.

Two things raise your risk. Being a woman raises it substantially, by a factor of several. And having thyroid antibodies before you start raises it, which is a reason to know whether you had them, and most people do not.

The onset clusters in the first two years, which is when nobody is looking, because in the first two years everyone is preoccupied with the psychiatric picture and any tiredness gets read as the illness settling.

10.2 Why This Is the Most Misattributed Problem in Psychiatry

Read these two lists.

Hypothyroidism: fatigue, weight gain, cold intolerance, constipation, slowed thinking, low mood, poor concentration, hair thinning, dry skin, reduced libido.

Depression: fatigue, weight gain or loss, low mood, poor concentration, slowed thinking, constipation, reduced libido.

There is one item on the first list that does not appear on the second in any useful way, and it is cold intolerance, which nobody asks about and which patients do not volunteer because being cold does not feel like a symptom.

That overlap is why this goes wrong so reliably. A patient on lithium reports low mood and tiredness. The clinician does what clinicians are trained to do, which is to think about mood. The lithium level is checked because that is the reflex. It is fine. So something is added, or a dose is changed, or a therapy referral is made, and the TSH sitting on a form from fourteen months ago is not looked at because nobody was thinking about the thyroid, because the patient came in with a mood complaint.

Frye and colleagues (1999) found something that makes this worse and more interesting. In lithium-maintained bipolar patients, lower free T4 was associated with greater mood instability and more depression, and this held within the normal range. Not in overt hypothyroidism. Within the range that would be reported as normal on your result. That finding is twenty-five years old and it has still not fully arrived in routine practice.

Which means "your thyroid is normal" may be doing the same work as "your level is fine" from Chapter 2.0. It is a statement about a number sitting inside a reference interval derived from a general population, and there is a real argument that the interval that matters for a person on lithium with an unstable mood is not the same interval.

10.3 The Other Gland Nobody Mentions

Calcium is on your monitoring form and nobody has explained it. Here is the explanation.

Lithium interferes with the parathyroid glands, four small glands sitting behind the thyroid whose entire job is regulating blood calcium. Lithium raises the threshold at which they decide there is enough calcium in circulation, so they keep secreting parathyroid hormone when they should have stopped, and blood calcium drifts up. Over years, the glands can enlarge.

Meehan and colleagues (2018) reviewed the prevalence and management of lithium-associated hypercalcemia; Albert and colleagues (2013) found it in a case-control study; Szalat and colleagues (2009) described the surgical end of it. Shine and colleagues (2015) found the calcium association in their laboratory data at least as clearly as the renal one.

The symptoms, and this is the point, are: tiredness, low mood, constipation, thirst, increased urination, aches, and difficulty concentrating.

Read that list again. Every single item on it is already explained by something else you have. The thirst and urination look like the nephrogenic diabetes insipidus from Chapter 9.0. The tiredness and low mood look like depression, or like hypothyroidism. The concentration problems look like the illness. There is no symptom of lithium-associated hypercalcemia that does not have three more available explanations, which is precisely why it is on the blood form, and precisely why it goes unchecked for years.

The following are composite cases.

Case A Joss, 39, had been on lithium for five years. At a routine review she mentioned that she was tired and had gained weight. Her clinician looked at her TSH from four months earlier, which was 5.8 and had been flagged as borderline by the lab and filed by nobody. He repeated it. It was 7.2. She started levothyroxine. Six weeks later her energy had returned and eight pounds had come off without her doing anything.

Case B Zennor, 41, had been on lithium for six years. She reported the same two things at her review. Her lithium level was checked and was fine. Her diagnosis was revised to bipolar depression with a poor response to lithium. Quetiapine was added, which sedated her and put on more weight, and then an antidepressant, which did not help. Twenty-two months later a locum GP ordered a thyroid function test for an unrelated reason and her TSH was 11.

The two women had the same problem. The difference was not diagnostic skill in any impressive sense. It was that one clinician looked at a piece of paper that already existed. Zennor's abnormal TSH was almost certainly present at her first review; nobody had ordered the test, so it was not on a screen, so it was not in anyone's mind. Two years of her life, two additional medications, and a revised diagnosis, all resting on a blood test that was never ordered.

One more thing belongs here, because it connects to the drug chapters. Thyroid and parathyroid effects are lithium effects. They are not mood stabiliser effects. Valproate does not do this. Lamotrigine does not do this. Carbamazepine does not do this, though it has its own endocrine mischief through enzyme induction, lowering vitamin D and affecting bone over years, which is a genuine long-term issue that almost nobody monitors for. If you are on lithium, the thyroid and calcium boxes are yours. If you are not, they are not, and a clinician checking them on you anyway is being thorough rather than worried.

10.4 What People Get Wrong About the Fix

"Hypothyroidism means I have to stop lithium." No. This is the most common misunderstanding and it causes real harm, because people who like their lithium hear the thyroid result as a threat and stop reporting symptoms. Lithium-induced hypothyroidism is treated by replacing the thyroid hormone, with levothyroxine, at a cost of one tablet and a few pounds a year. The lithium continues. This is one of the few places in this entire book where the answer is genuinely easy.

"Treating the thyroid is admitting the lithium failed." No. It is a manageable side effect being managed. Nobody thinks a person on a statin has failed at cholesterol.

"My TSH is in range so my thyroid is not the problem." Possibly not true, per Frye. Worth asking about free T4 specifically if your mood is unstable and your TSH is drifting upward inside the range, particularly if the drift is your own drift rather than a population deviation.

"Hypercalcemia is a serious diagnosis." Usually not. Mild lithium-associated hypercalcemia is often managed by monitoring and by treating what it is causing. Occasionally it needs a parathyroid operation. Mostly it needs somebody to have noticed it.

The following account is a composite, with details changed for anonymity.

Merritt, whose eight months of depression inside a therapeutic lithium range opened Chapter 1.0, is worth returning to, because the story did not end where that chapter left it.

His TSH came back elevated, he started levothyroxine, and he improved, though not completely, which is why lamotrigine was added later. That was the account given at nine months and it was accurate as far as it went.

What it left out was the year that followed. His TSH came back into range. His energy returned. The eleven pounds did not come off, because by then he had been sedentary for a year and the weight had acquired its own momentum, which is a thing weight does and which Chapter 11.0 has more to say about. And he remained, in his own description, about a third short of where he had been.

His question, which he asked once and then stopped asking, was whether the eight months had cost him something permanent. Nobody could answer it. The honest position is that we do not know whether prolonged untreated hypothyroidism in a bipolar patient leaves a residue, and the studies that would answer it have not been done.

What Merritt did with the not-knowing is what most people do. He got on with it. He also, four years later, still checks his own TSH result on the patient portal before his appointments, which his psychiatrist finds slightly unusual and which is, if you look at it clearly, the entirely rational response of a man who lost eight months because a piece of paper went unread.

> **Teaching Point:** *The cost of a missed thyroid result is not only the interval of illness. It includes the weight, the deconditioning, and the loss of trust, none of which reverse when the TSH does.*
>
> **Teaching Point:** *Patients who check their own results are usually described as anxious. Often they are described as anxious by the service that gave them the reason.*

10.5 Pulling the Threads

Start here: lithium interferes with the thyroid in a large minority of people and with the parathyroid glands in a smaller one, and both effects produce tiredness, weight gain, low mood, and poor concentration. That is not an incidental overlap. It is the central problem, because those four symptoms are also the illness the lithium is treating.

Build on that: since the symptoms cannot distinguish the causes, and the clinician's observation cannot distinguish the causes, the distinction rests entirely on a blood test. Not on skill, not on listening, not on the therapeutic relationship. On a test being ordered and then read. Joss got better in six weeks and Zennor lost twenty-two months, and the whole of the difference was a piece of paper that one clinician opened.

Then add this: the test being on the guideline does not mean the test gets done, and the test being done does not mean the result gets read, and Chapter 2.0 already established that lithium monitoring falls into the gap between services. Which means the last line of defense against the most reversible cause of your depression is a person with no medical training who knows to look at their own TSH.

That is a bad system. It is also, for the moment, the system. So: know your last TSH, know its date, and know the one symptom on the hypothyroid list that is not on the depression list. If you have been quietly cold since August and nobody has asked you about it, that is worth a sentence at your next appointment, and it is worth more than everything else in this chapter put together.

Chapter 11.0 takes the weight that has been accumulating quietly in the background of the last three chapters and asks the question nobody asks, which is not how to lose it but what actually put it there.

Chapter 11.0: Four Reasons You Gained Weight

Bellamy and Cypress both started lithium in the same March, at the same clinic, at similar doses, and both had gained around 30 pounds by Christmas. Same drug, same interval, almost the same number on the scale. Eighteen months later Bellamy had lost 24 of them and Cypress had gained another 11 and stopped taking lithium entirely, which was followed within the year by the first manic episode she had had since her twenties. Neither woman ate differently from the other in any way that would show up on a food diary. Neither exercised more than the other. What separated them was a question that took four minutes and that only one of them was ever asked.

11.1 The Problem Is That It Is Not One Problem

Weight gain is the most common reason people stop taking mood stabilisers, and it is the least well handled thing in this book.

The reason it is handled badly is not that clinicians do not care. It is that "weight gain" gets treated as a single event with a single cause, and it is not. It is at least five different physiological processes that happen to converge on the same number, and they respond to entirely different interventions. Treating them as one thing produces the standard advice, which is diet and exercise, delivered with a slight air of disappointment, to a person whose problem is fluid retention or an underactive thyroid.

Torrent and colleagues (2008), reviewing weight gain in bipolar disorder, made the point that gets lost in every appointment: the pharmacological contribution is real, it is separable, and it varies enormously by agent. Vendsborg and colleagues (1976) established the lithium association almost fifty years ago. Fagiolini and colleagues (2002) documented the scale of obesity in bipolar I populations and how much of it accumulates during treatment.

So the useful question is not how to lose it. It is: which of the five is yours?

11.2 The Five, and How to Tell Them Apart

One: thirst met with calories. Lithium is a salt. It makes you thirsty, and the nephrogenic diabetes insipidus described in Chapter 9.0 makes you thirstier still. What you quench that thirst with is the entire question. Three liters a day of full-sugar cola is around 1,200 calories that did not exist in your life before March. Three liters of water is none.

This is the mechanism that should be addressed before you ever take the first tablet, and virtually never is. The right moment to ask someone what they drink when they are thirsty is the day you write the prescription, not the day they have gained two stone. Ask afterwards and you are asking someone to change a habit they have built under physiological pressure. Ask before and it is a preference.

How to recognize it: the gain is gradual, tracks with the thirst, and you can find it in what you drink if you are honest about a whole day.

Two: fluid. Lithium causes sodium and water retention, and the NDI physiology contributes. Some people put on weight very fast at the start, and fast weight is not fat. Adipose tissue cannot accumulate at that rate. It is water.

This one has an actual treatment, and it is one of the few genuinely satisfying facts in this chapter. Batlle and colleagues (1985), in the New England Journal of Medicine, showed that amiloride relieved the polyuria of long-term lithium therapy. Amiloride is preferred over thiazide diuretics for a specific reason:

it does not usually raise lithium levels, whereas thiazides raise them by 50 to 100 percent, which Chapter 7.0 called a dose doubling arriving through a blood pressure prescription. Amiloride can occasionally shift a level too, so it warrants a check. But there is a drug for this, most people are never offered it, and the reason is that nobody categorized their weight gain as fluid in the first place.

How to recognize it: rapid onset, early, sometimes with puffiness in the ankles or fingers, and disproportionate to anything you have eaten.

Three: the thyroid. Chapter 10.0 spent 2,000 words on this and the summary is one sentence: slow weight accrual over months, with fatigue and feeling cold, on lithium, is hypothyroidism until a TSH says otherwise.

How to recognize it: slow, months, with tiredness, with cold, and it does not respond to eating less.

Four: carbohydrate craving. This one is real, it is reported consistently, and it is the one with the worst answers. A proportion of people on lithium describe a specific pull toward bread, sugar, and baked goods that they did not have before. Chen and Silverstone (1990) examined lithium and weight gain and appetite change is a consistent thread through that literature. Managing it is genuinely difficult and I am not going to pretend otherwise. What helps is knowing in advance that it is coming, because a craving you were warned about is a different experience from a craving that arrives as evidence of your own weakness.

How to recognize it: you know. This is the one people can identify immediately when it is described to them.

Five: the confounders, and there are two. The first is that atypical-feature bipolar depression independently produces increased appetite and weight gain. If you are depressed with atypical features, you would be gaining weight without any drug at all, and the lithium is getting blamed for the illness. The second is that most people are not on lithium alone. Olanzapine and quetiapine cause substantially more weight gain than lithium does, and valproate is no lightweight either. If you are on lithium plus quetiapine and you have gained 30 pounds, the arithmetic almost certainly does not favor the lithium, and stopping the lithium would be solving the wrong problem.

Which is worth stating in a sentence, because it is the practical heart of this chapter: lamotrigine is essentially weight-neutral. Bowden and colleagues (2006) examined the impact of lamotrigine and lithium on weight in obese and non-obese patients with bipolar I and found lamotrigine did not produce the gain. If your regimen contains one agent driving your weight and one that is not, the question is which one to move, and it is not automatically the one with the blood tests.

11.3 What Happened to Bellamy

The following are composite cases.

Case A Bellamy raised the weight at her nine-month review. Her clinician asked, as the first question rather than the last: what do you drink when you are thirsty, and how much? The answer was around two and a half liters of orange squash a day, made strong, because she was thirsty constantly and water made her feel sick. That is somewhere around 800 calories nobody had counted. Her TSH was also checked and was mildly raised. Both were addressed. Over eighteen months she lost 24 pounds and stayed on lithium.

Case B Cypress raised the weight at her nine-month review too. She was advised to look at her diet and to try to be more active, which was reasonable advice and which she followed. She kept a food diary for six weeks. It showed nothing remarkable, because the diary had a column for food and not for drink. Her weight continued upward. At eighteen months she stopped the lithium without discussing it, having concluded that the drug was making her ill and that nobody was going to help.

The contrast is not about effort. Cypress tried considerably harder than Bellamy did; she kept the diary, she walked. The contrast is that one of them was asked a question with a mechanism behind it and the other was given advice with a moral shape to it. And the food diary is the detail that says everything, because a food diary is an instrument designed to find calories in food, given to a woman whose calories were in a jug.

11.4 Running the Differential

The following is a composite case; identifying details have been changed.

Background Cypress returned to services fourteen months after her manic episode, restarted on lithium, and 41 pounds heavier than she had been in the March she started it the first time.

Presentation She opened the appointment by saying that she would take the lithium and that she was not prepared to gain more weight, and that if it came to a choice she already knew which way she would go. That is not resistance and it should not be recorded as such. It is a person stating a constraint.

Analysis This time the workup was done properly and it took eleven minutes.

Drink: two liters of squash a day. Present. Speed of the original gain: 14 pounds in the first ten weeks, which is faster than fat accumulates. Fluid, at least in part. Present. TSH: 6.1. Present. Craving: she described wanting bread in a way she never had before. Present. Other agents: she was on quetiapine 200 mg at night for sleep, added during the manic episode and never reviewed. Atypical depression: her depressive episodes had always involved oversleeping and eating more. Present.

Six mechanisms. All six. Which is exactly why the standard advice had failed, and it is also why "which one is yours" turns out, for many people, to be the wrong question. Sometimes the answer is all of them.

Intervention The squash was swapped for water with cordial, sugar-free, which she loathed and did anyway. Levothyroxine was started. Amiloride was added for the fluid, with a lithium level at two weeks. The quetiapine was tapered over four months and replaced with nothing, and her sleep was worse for about six weeks and then was not.

Outcome At two years she had lost 29 of the 41 pounds. She remains on lithium. She still wants bread.

> **Teaching Point:** *Five mechanisms are not a menu. In a person who has been on a complex regimen for years, most of them are usually present simultaneously.*
>
> **Teaching Point:** *Nothing in that eleven-minute workup required specialist knowledge. It required a list.*
>
> **Teaching Point:** *"I would rather relapse than gain more weight" is a statement of the patient's actual utility function. Arguing with it wastes the appointment. Working within it produces a plan.*

11.5 Settling the Account

Cypress lost a year of her life to a manic episode that followed a decision to stop lithium, and the decision to stop lithium followed eighteen months of gaining weight that nobody had explained to her. It is tempting to draw a line straight through that and call the weight gain the cause of the relapse. That would be too neat, and it would let the wrong thing off the hook.

The weight gain did not cause the relapse. What caused the relapse was that she was given advice with a moral shape when she needed a question with a mechanism behind it, and the difference between those two things is about four minutes, and nobody had four minutes.

Her second workup found six mechanisms operating at once in a woman who had been told, in effect, to eat less. Every one of the six was identifiable with information that already existed. The speed of her original gain was in her notes. The TSH was orderable. The quetiapine was on her repeat prescription. The squash was in her kitchen and would have been in the room too, if anyone had asked.

So the account here does not settle in favor of better willpower or better drugs. It settles on a much duller finding, which is that the most common reason people abandon an effective medication is a side effect that nobody bothered to take apart into its components. Bellamy stayed on lithium because someone asked her what she drank. That is the whole intervention. It is not clever and it is barely medicine, and it is the difference between the two women in this chapter.

Ask what you drink. Look at how fast it came on. Check the thyroid. Count the other drugs. And if you are the person in the chair rather than the person with the prescription pad, you can run all four of those yourself, before the appointment, on the back of an envelope.

Chapter 12.0 turns to the decision where the stakes stop being about you.

Chapter 12.0: Pregnancy and the Real Numbers

There is no safe option, and anybody who offers you one is either not telling you the truth or has not understood the question. Every path available to a woman with bipolar disorder who wants a child carries risk. Taking the drug carries risk to the baby. Stopping the drug carries risk to the mother, and through her to the baby, and the risk of stopping is substantially larger than most people are told and considerably better documented than the risk of continuing. The field's honest position is that this is a choice between quantified harms, made with incomplete information, in a body that will not wait for better evidence. What follows is the best account of the numbers that currently exists. It will not make the decision easy. It should make it yours.

12.1 The Disagreement, Stated Fairly

The two positions are not held by fools and they are not caricatures of each other.

The first says: pregnancy is nine months, the exposure window that matters most is the first trimester, and the fetus cannot consent. Where a drug is known to cause malformation or developmental harm, the default should be to stop, and the burden of proof should sit on continuing. Psychiatric risk is real but it is a risk to an adult who can be monitored, supported, and hospitalized if necessary. Teratogenic damage is permanent and it happens to someone else.

The second says: that framing treats maternal illness as an inconvenience rather than a danger, and it is factually wrong about the size of the risks. Bipolar disorder in the perinatal period is not low mood. It is one of the highest-risk periods for severe psychiatric illness in the whole of medicine, and the leading causes of maternal death in the year after birth in high-income countries include suicide. Removing effective treatment from a woman at the exact moment her risk peaks is not a neutral act, and calling it "stopping" rather than "an intervention with its own harms" obscures what is being done.

I have a position on this and I will state it rather than hide it: the second argument is closer to right, and the reason is that only one side of this ledger has been counted properly for most of the last forty years. But it is not a rout, and the valproate story in Chapter 4.0 is what happens when the second argument wins for too long without scrutiny.

12.2 The Case for Caution, With Its Numbers

Valproate. The strongest version of the cautious argument is simply valproate, and the argument wins. Roughly three to five percent neural tube defects, the highest major congenital malformation rate of eight antiepileptic drugs in the EURAP registry (Tomson et al., 2018), and 30 to 40 percent neurodevelopmental disorder in exposed children (Meador et al., 2013; Christensen et al., 2013). There is no reading of that data on which valproate is acceptable in a pregnancy that could be avoided. This is not a debate. It is the settled part.

Carbamazepine. Roughly one percent neural tube defect risk (Jentink et al., 2010). Real, an order of magnitude below valproate, and enough to make it a poor first choice.

Lithium. Here the argument gets interesting, because lithium is where the cautious position has historically been strongest and where it has most clearly been wrong.

In 1974, Nora and colleagues reported a striking association between lithium and Ebstein's anomaly, a malformation of the tricuspid valve. The data came from the International Register of Lithium Babies, a voluntary reporting scheme, and the resulting estimate suggested exposed children were something like 400 times more likely to have the defect. That number entered the textbooks and it stayed there for two decades.

It was wrong. Voluntary registers collect the cases people think are worth reporting, which means they collect the disasters and miss the healthy babies entirely. Cohen and colleagues (1994) reevaluated the risk and found it far smaller. Fornaro and colleagues (2020), pooling the subsequent literature, found smaller still.

Then Patorno and colleagues (2017) did the study that settled it, in the New England Journal of Medicine, across 1,325,563 Medicaid pregnancies. Cardiac malformations occurred in 2.41 per 100 live births among lithium-exposed infants, 1.15 per 100 among unexposed, and 1.39 per 100 among lamotrigine-exposed. The adjusted risk ratio was 1.65, with a confidence interval from 1.02 to 2.68. For the right ventricular outflow tract defects, which is the Ebstein's family: 0.60 per 100 exposed against 0.18 per 100 unexposed, adjusted risk ratio 2.66, confidence interval 1.00 to 7.06.

Translate that into the sentence that matters. If your baseline risk of a cardiac malformation is about 1.15 percent, first-trimester lithium takes it to roughly 1.9 percent. Not 400-fold. Under one percentage point of absolute risk. Munk-Olsen and colleagues (2018), in an international collaborative meta-analysis of six cohorts, arrived at a consistent picture.

The risk is real and it is dose-related. It is also, if you were told the 1970s number, roughly two orders of magnitude smaller than what you are carrying around in your head.

Lamotrigine. The comparator with the least signal. Tomson's registry data puts it lowest of the eight. Hernández-Díaz and colleagues (2024), examining autism risk after prenatal exposure to topiramate, valproate, and lamotrigine, did not find the lamotrigine signal that the valproate data would have predicted if this were a class effect. It is not a class effect. It is a valproate effect.

12.3 The Case for Continuing, With Its Numbers

Here is the number that almost nobody is given, and it is the largest number in this chapter.

Viguera and colleagues (2007a) followed 89 women with bipolar disorder prospectively through pregnancy, all euthymic at conception, comparing those who continued mood stabilisers with those who discontinued. Across the whole cohort, 71 percent had at least one recurrence during the pregnancy. Split by what they did: recurrence was 85.5 percent in the women who stopped and 37 percent in the women who continued. The women who discontinued spent over 40 percent of the pregnancy in an episode, against 8.8 percent of those who continued. And rapid discontinuation was worse than tapering, by a factor of about 11 in median time to recurrence.

Eighty-five percent against 37. Set that next to the 0.95 percentage point adjusted increment in cardiac malformation from Patorno and notice that these two numbers are almost never presented on the same page, and that the smaller one is the one everybody has heard of.

Then the postpartum, which is worse. Wesseloo and colleagues (2016), pooling 37 studies covering 5,700 deliveries, found an overall postpartum relapse risk across high-risk women of 35 percent, and a relapse risk of 37 percent in women with bipolar disorder specifically. Severe episodes were less common: 17 percent in bipolar disorder, 29 percent in women with a history of postpartum psychosis. Postpartum psychosis is a psychiatric emergency with a real mortality, it comes on fast, and bipolar disorder is its single largest risk factor.

The number in that paper that should end the argument is a different one. Among women with bipolar disorder, postpartum relapse was 66 percent in those who went through pregnancy medication free and 23 percent in those who took prophylactic medication. Sixty-six against 23. That is not a subtle effect and it is not a contested one.

Bergink and colleagues (2012) showed that prophylaxis, meaning lithium started immediately after delivery in women at high risk, substantially reduced that. That finding has a consequence people find counterintuitive: for some women the most important lithium decision is not about pregnancy at all. It is about the twenty-four hours after the birth.

The following account is a composite, with details changed for anonymity.

Fable, whose benign rash in week six opened Chapter 3.0 and who reached her target lamotrigine dose in week eight, became pregnant four years later.

Her preconception appointment happened, unusually, before conception, because she asked for it. That fact alone put her in a small minority. Most of these conversations happen with a positive test already in hand, which removes the first trimester from the discussion entirely, since by the time most women know they are pregnant the neural tube has already closed.

The plan was straightforward because her drug was the least bad one in this chapter. She stayed on lamotrigine. Her dose was monitored, which surprised her, because Chapter 3.0 had told her lamotrigine needs no blood levels, and in pregnancy that stops being true. Lamotrigine clearance rises substantially through pregnancy, sometimes to the point where a woman on a stable dose is functionally under-treated by the third trimester, and the dose has to climb to keep up, and then come back down after delivery or she becomes toxic.

Nobody had told her that. It is not in the leaflet. She found out because her perinatal psychiatrist knew it, and she has since said the thing that a lot of women in this situation say, which is that she cannot stop thinking about the version of herself who did not get referred to a perinatal service and who spent her third trimester wondering why the drug had stopped working.

She had a boy. She had a difficult six weeks postpartum and did not have an episode.

> **Teaching Point:** *The pharmacology of every drug in this book changes during pregnancy. A stable dose is not a stable exposure.*
>
> **Teaching Point:** *Preconception, not postconception, is when this conversation is worth having, and the interval between them contains the entire first trimester.*

12.4 Where the Evidence Runs Out

Four honest gaps.

Nobody knows what the untreated illness does to the fetus. We measure drug exposure against unexposed controls. We do not have good data on what a manic episode in the second trimester, or a severe depression with poor nutrition and no antenatal care, does to a developing child. That is not a small omission. It means one entire column of the ledger is estimated rather than measured, and it is systematically the column that favors continuing.

The lithium dose relationship is not well characterized. Higher exposure looks worse. Where the threshold sits, and whether a woman at 0.5 mmol/L carries meaningfully less risk than one at 0.9, is not answerable with current data.

Breastfeeding on lithium is genuinely unsettled. The historical position was that it was contraindicated. Viguera and colleagues (2007b) measured lithium in breast milk and in nursing infants and found the exposures lower than expected. Imaz and colleagues (2019), reviewing the lactation studies, found the evidence thin but not alarming. The current position in most services is that it is possible in a healthy, term infant with monitoring, and that it is a decision rather than a prohibition. Anyone telling you it is definitely fine or definitely not is going beyond the data.

The paternal question from Chapter 4.0 remains open. One observational signal, an evidence review finding no clear effect, and a regulatory position already revised once.

12.5 The Same Decision, Twice

The following are composite cases.

Case A Solstice, 31, bipolar I, one prior admission for mania, stable on lithium for six years. She planned a pregnancy, tapered lithium slowly over three months before conceiving, remained off it through the first trimester, restarted at the beginning of the second, and had lithium at delivery with careful attention to hydration in labor. She had a girl. No episode.

Case B Tatum, 33, bipolar I, three prior admissions including one postpartum psychosis after her first child. She stayed on lithium throughout, including the first trimester. Her fetal cardiac scan at 20 weeks was normal. She had a boy. No episode.

Both women were right, and the reason is the sentence that should be printed on the front of every perinatal psychiatry service in the country: the decision is not determined by the drug. It is determined by the history.

Solstice had one episode, years ago, and a low postpartum risk, which made a first-trimester gap a reasonable price for removing the cardiac increment. Tatum had already had postpartum psychosis, which put her risk of a severe postpartum episode at something close to 29 percent, and a first-trimester gap would have bought her a 0.75 percentage point reduction in cardiac malformation risk at the cost of destabilizing the drug she would need most in the twenty-four hours after delivery. For Tatum, the arithmetic did not just favor continuing. It was not close.

12.6 The Open Questions

The number that should be sitting in your head at the end of this chapter is not 2.41 per 100. It is not 0.60 per 100 either, and it is certainly not 400-fold, which was never real.

It is 85.5 percent against 37, from Viguera, and 66 against 23, from Wesseloo. Those are the numbers that describe what happens to the woman, they are two orders of magnitude larger than the ones that get quoted at her, and they are almost never in the room.

Which raises the question this chapter has been building toward, and it is a real one rather than a rhetorical one. Given that both columns of this ledger have been measurable for at least fifteen years, why is it that almost every woman with bipolar disorder who becomes pregnant can recite the Ebstein's story, and almost none of them has ever heard the discontinuation figure?

I do not think the answer is that clinicians are careless. I think the answer is that the two risks are not felt to be the same kind of thing. A malformation caused by a drug a doctor prescribed is an act. A relapse caused by a drug a doctor stopped is an event. The first appears in a coroner's language and the second appears in a discharge summary, and the entire architecture of medicolegal caution points one way.

That asymmetry is not a fact about your baby. It is a fact about liability. And once you can see it, you can ask the question that actually gets you a good conversation, which is not "is lithium safe in pregnancy" but: what is my risk of relapse if I stop, what is my risk if I do not, and can you show me both numbers, on the same page, before I decide?

Chapter 13.0 changes the reader. Everything so far has been written to the person taking the tablet. The next one is for the person watching.

Chapter 13.0: What Your Family Should Watch

A man whose wife has bipolar disorder once said that the hardest part was not the crises. It was the ordinary Tuesdays, when she was slightly off and he did not know whether he was noticing something or inventing it, and whether saying anything would help her or insult her. He had been right, he said, about four times out of five over twenty years. He had also been wrong once, badly, in a way she had not forgiven quickly. And so he had learned to say nothing until he was certain, which meant, he said, that he had learned to say nothing until it was too late to matter.

13.1 This Chapter Is for You

If you are the person with the diagnosis, hand this over. Read it too, but hand it over.

Everything in this book so far has been addressed to the person taking the tablet. This chapter is addressed to whoever is standing next to them: a partner, a parent, an adult child, a friend who has been around long enough to know what the normal version looks like.

There is a reason you get a chapter, and it is not sentiment. It is that on the specific question of medication side effects and early relapse, you have better data than the clinician does, and you frequently have better data than the patient does. The clinician sees fifteen minutes every four months. You see a Tuesday. And several of the things this book is about, coarse tremor, thyroid slowing, the first two days of a manic prodrome, are conditions in which the affected person's ability to assess themselves is precisely the faculty being affected.

That is not a metaphor. Chapter 8.0 described Zephyr, who was unsteady and slurring and genuinely believed he was fine. He was not lying. Lithium at 1.9 mmol/L had taken away the instrument he would have needed to notice.

So you are not a spare part in this. You are the early warning system, and nobody has ever trained you.

13.2 The Four Things That Look Like Each Other

Here is where you will go wrong, and it is worth being specific, because "watch for changes" is useless advice.

Lithium tremor versus anxiety. A fine, fast tremor in the hands is a normal lithium side effect and it means nothing. Roughly a third of people on lithium have one. It is not distress and it is not a warning, and if you read it as nervousness you will spend years worrying about the wrong thing. What matters is a change in its character: coarser, slower, larger, more like a shake than a buzz. Learn what their normal tremor looks like now, this week, while everything is fine. That baseline is the single most useful thing you can acquire from this chapter and it takes ten seconds.

Sedation versus depression. Someone on olanzapine or quetiapine who sleeps eleven hours and is flat until noon may be sedated rather than depressed. The distinguishing feature is not mood, because both look flat. It is interest. A sedated person who is woken and gets going is often fine by two in the afternoon and wants things. A depressed person is flat at two as well, and does not want anything, and would not want it even if they had the energy.

Thyroid flattening versus a depressive episode. Chapter 10.0 made this case at length. Tiredness, weight gain, slowness, low mood, and being cold. That last one is the giveaway and it is the one that never gets mentioned, because being cold does not feel like a symptom to the person who is cold. If they have been putting a jumper on in a room where you are comfortable, and this is new, that is a piece of clinical information and you are the only person who has it.

Prodrome versus a bad week. The hardest one. Everyone has bad weeks. What distinguishes the beginning of an episode is usually not intensity but pattern: sleep going first and going without tiredness following it, speech quickening, projects starting, spending, a specific kind of certainty. Or on the other side: withdrawal, cancelled plans, a flattening of the voice on the phone.

The honest thing to say about the fourth one is that you will get it wrong sometimes. So will they. So will their psychiatrist. The goal is not accuracy. It is a system in which being wrong is cheap.

There is a fifth thing, and it sits outside that list because it is not a confusion. It is the one where you are simply the only person in the room.

Lithium toxicity, described in Chapter 8.0, is a condition you will identify from outside and they will not identify from inside. The three signs are unsteadiness, slurred speech, and a tremor that has changed character, usually alongside something that has dried them out: a stomach bug, a hot week, a new tablet from a GP. If you see those and they tell you they are fine, they are not lying to you and they are not being stubborn. The drug has affected the faculty they would need to answer you accurately.

The same is true, in a smaller way, of carbamazepine's hyponatremia. Vagueness and a fall in someone on carbamazepine is a blood test, not a conversation.

For those two, the assessment is yours and the decision has to be yours, which is exactly why the next section exists.

13.3 The Agreement, Made While Well

This is the mechanism, and everything else in the chapter is decoration around it.

Chapter 8.0 described Zephyr's daughter overriding him at his kitchen table, and the reason she was able to do it: eighteen months earlier, when he was well, he had told her to. He had said, out loud, that if she ever thought he was toxic she should act and ignore whatever he said at the time. He had felt slightly theatrical saying it. It turned out to be the entire mechanism.

You need one of those. Not a vague understanding. A conversation, held on a day when nothing is wrong, with a small number of specific things in it.

What am I allowed to say, and how? Agree the words in advance. "I've noticed you haven't slept much this week" is a sentence about an observation. "You're getting high again" is a sentence about a person. The first one is answerable and the second one is a fight. Pick the sentence together, now, and then you are not choosing it under pressure.

What are the two or three signs that matter most for you? Not a list of thirty. Two or three, specific to this person, drawn from what happened last time. For most people the first is sleep. Write them down.

What happens when I say it? This is the part that gets skipped and it is the part that makes the rest work. If the agreement is only "I will tell you," then every warning is a confrontation with no exit. If the agreement is "I will tell you, and you will phone the service within 48 hours, and that is all that happens," then the warning has somewhere to go and it costs almost nothing to be wrong.

What is the override? The narrow, explicit, named circumstance in which you act regardless of what they say at the time. Unsteady and slurring on lithium. That is Zephyr's. It should be as specific as that, and it should be given, not taken.

Write it on one sheet. Appendix F is laid out for it.

13.4 Two Families, One Signal

The following are composite cases.

Case A Indigo's husband noticed she had been up until three for four nights, and that she was not tired. He said the agreed sentence: I've noticed you haven't slept much this week. She said she was fine and was irritated. He said the second agreed sentence, which was that he was going to hold her to the 48 hours. She phoned her service on day two, out of a sense of obligation rather than concern, and a small medication change was made. Nothing dramatic happened. There was no episode. She has never fully accepted that there would have been one, and she may be right, and it does not matter.

Case B Fallon's mother noticed the same thing in her daughter and said nothing for eleven days, because the last time she had raised it, three years earlier, Fallon had accused her of never believing she was well and they had not spoken for a month. By the time she said something, Fallon had spent four thousand pounds and resigned from her job by email at four in the morning.

The mother had not failed to notice. She noticed on day two. What she lacked was permission, and what she had instead was a memory of what it cost her last time. Eleven days of silence was not neglect. It was a rational response to a system in which raising a concern was expensive and being wrong was catastrophic to the relationship.

The difference between the two families was not vigilance, and it was not love, and it was certainly not insight. It was that one of them had held a fifteen-minute conversation on a good day and the other had not.

13.5 Your Own Limits

Three things, and they belong here rather than in a self-care appendix.

You will be resented. Sometimes by the person you are protecting, sometimes for years, and being right does not exempt you from it. Indigo has never conceded that her husband prevented an episode. He has had to be all right with that, and being all right with it is not the same as it being fair.

You are not the treatment. You are a monitor with a good sensor and no medical training and no capacity to intervene, and the whole of the agreement in 13.3 is designed to hand the problem to someone with more power than you as quickly as possible. If you find yourself managing rather than reporting, that is a sign that the service has quietly transferred a job to you that it should be doing.

And your own capacity is finite in a way that nobody will ask about. Nobody schedules a review for you. There is no six-monthly appointment for the person doing the noticing. If you are exhausted, that is information about the arrangement rather than a failing in you, and the arrangement is the thing that needs changing.

13.6 What to Carry Forward

The man at the start of this chapter said he had learned to say nothing until he was certain, which meant he had learned to say nothing until it was too late to matter. I have thought about that sentence a great deal and I think he had diagnosed his situation exactly, and had drawn the wrong conclusion from it.

He was not wrong that certainty comes late. It does. By the time you are sure, the sleep has gone and the money is spent. The error was in thinking that certainty was the threshold, and he thought that because the cost of being wrong in his marriage was enormous. Twenty years, one bad mistake, not forgiven quickly.

Which means the problem was never his judgment. His judgment was excellent; four out of five over two decades is better than most clinicians manage with the same information. The problem was that the price of a false alarm in that house was set so high that a man with an 80 percent hit rate could not afford to use it.

That is the thing to carry forward, and it is the whole chapter. The agreement in 13.3 does one job, which is to bring the cost of being wrong down to something like a phone call. Once a false alarm is cheap, you can act on suspicion instead of proof, and suspicion arrives on day two rather than day eleven. You are not trying to become more accurate. You are already accurate enough. You are trying to build a house in which being wrong is survivable.

Have the conversation on a good day. Agree the sentence. Agree the 48 hours. Name the override out loud, and make sure it is given rather than taken. It takes fifteen minutes and it is worth more than every appointment either of you will attend this year.

Chapter 14.0 goes back to the person taking the tablet, and to the part of this that no leaflet mentions at all, which is what it is like to do this for thirty years.

Chapter 14.0: Living On It

The pill organizer is the kind with seven compartments and a hinged lid for each day, and it cost about four pounds. Xael has been filling one every Sunday evening for nineteen years. He does it at the kitchen table, usually while the kettle boils, and it takes ninety seconds. There is nothing remarkable about the object at all. What is remarkable, if you think about it for a moment, is the arithmetic sitting inside it: nineteen years, fifty-two Sundays a year, close to a thousand of them. Nobody prepares you for the thousand. The leaflet covers the tablet. The clinic covers the level. There is no appointment, anywhere in the system, at which somebody sits down with you and discusses what it is like to do this until you are old.

14.1 The Problem With Decades

Every chapter so far has been about an event. A blood test. A rash in week six. A holiday that went wrong. A pregnancy. Events have edges, and edges are what medicine is good at.

The thing that actually characterizes long-term mood stabiliser treatment is not any of those. It is duration. It is the accumulation of ordinary Sundays, and the way a set of small compromises that were entirely reasonable at 26 become a shape you are living inside at 45 without ever having agreed to it.

The literature on this is thin, and the thinness is itself informative. We have hundreds of trials of efficacy over eighteen months. We have Baldessarini and Tondo (2000) showing lithium response holds stable over three decades, which is genuinely reassuring and answers a question about the drug. What we do not have is much of anything about the person: what it costs to organize your fluid intake around your kidney for twenty years, what it does to your sense of yourself to have a shelf in your bathroom that is not negotiable, what happens to a marriage in which one person has an agreement about overriding the other.

Those are not soft questions. Scott and Pope (2002) found nonadherence with mood stabilisers to be common, and the predictors were not what a pharmacology-first view would predict. Jamison and colleagues (1979), in a study that is now nearly fifty years old and has not been bettered, asked patients and physicians what they thought about lithium and found the two groups were not troubled by the same things at all. Patients were preoccupied by what the drug did to their sense of themselves. Physicians were preoccupied by levels and side effects.

Which means when people stop taking these drugs, and roughly half of them do at some point, the reason is often sitting in a category that nobody in the clinic has a form for.

14.2 The Practical Problems Nobody Briefs You On

Travel. Heat is a lithium event, as Chapter 7.0 established, and a holiday is a heat event with alcohol in it. Time zones matter less than people fear: a lithium dose taken six hours out of position for a week is not a crisis, and shifting gradually is fine. What matters more is the hand luggage rule, which is that your tablets travel with you and never in the hold, and the pharmacy rule, which is that lithium is not available everywhere and is called different things where it is. Carry a note with the generic name and the dose. Carry more than you need.

Work and shifts. Rotating night shifts are, for a person with bipolar disorder, an occupational hazard in the literal sense, and it has almost nothing to do with the tablet. Sleep disruption is the single most reliable trigger there is. The drug will not protect you from a rota that is deranging your circadian rhythm three weeks in four, and no dose adjustment substitutes for a different rota.

Disclosure. Nobody can tell you whether to disclose at work, and anyone who gives you a confident answer is generalizing from their own situation. The narrow, practical point is separable from the political one: somebody at your workplace should know that you take a medication that requires you to drink and to be careful in heat, and that is a much smaller disclosure than a diagnosis.

Surgery, dental work, and scans. Chapter 7.0 named this and it belongs here too because it recurs across decades. An anesthetist needs to know about lithium; the interactions with neuromuscular blocking agents are real and well described in the anesthetic literature (Peck et al., 2010). Being starved of fluids from midnight raises your level. Contrast for imaging concerns your kidney. None of these people will ask you a question that gets the answer.

Ageing. This is the one that gets least attention and is changing fastest. The kidney handles lithium less efficiently with age, so the same dose delivers a higher level in a 72-year-old than it did in the same person at 40. Other medications accumulate, most of them capable of shifting the level. Rej and colleagues (2012, 2015) reviewed lithium and renal function in older adults, and the ISBD task force on older-age bipolar disorder (Sajatovic et al., 2015) set out how thoroughly this population has been understudied. Shulman and colleagues (2019) had to run a Delphi survey of expert opinion on maintenance lithium in older adults, which is what a field does when it has no data.

The practical consequence: if you are over 65 on lithium, your dose probably needs to come down, your monitoring probably needs to be more frequent than six-monthly, and Chapter 9.0's kidney arithmetic looks meaningfully different for you than it does for a 30-year-old. Almost nobody is told this at the point it becomes true, because there is no appointment at which a person turns 65 in psychiatry.

14.3 The Pivot Is a Different Question

Here is what changed my thinking about this, and it did not come from a trial.

The field's approach to long-term treatment has been to optimize the drug: right agent, right level, right monitoring. That is necessary and this book has spent thirteen chapters on it. What it does not do is address the thing that actually makes people stop, which is not a side effect but a relationship.

Mogens Schou, who spent his career establishing lithium's maintenance efficacy, did something in 1979 that almost nobody has followed up. He studied artistic productivity in people on lithium prophylaxis, because artists kept telling him the drug had taken something from them. He took the complaint seriously enough to investigate it rather than reframing it as poor insight. What he found was mixed and more interesting than either camp wanted: most continued to work, some were more productive because they were less ill, and a minority reported a real loss.

Judd and colleagues (1977) had done something adjacent, giving lithium to healthy volunteers and measuring what happened to their affect and personality. The volunteers reported feeling less able, more lethargic, and duller.

So when a patient tells you lithium has flattened them, there is a small, old, entirely legitimate literature that says: possibly yes. That is not the response most people get. Most people get told it is the illness, or the depression, or that they are noticing the absence of hypomania and misdescribing it as loss.

Sometimes that reframe is correct. The point is that it is offered as though it were always correct, and it is not, and the fifty-year-old data says so.

The cognitive question has a similar shape. Wingo and colleagues (2009) meta-analyzed the effects of lithium on cognitive performance and found small effects on psychomotor speed and verbal memory, statistically real, of a size most people would not notice, and considerably smaller than the effect of being unwell. Pachet and Wisniewski (2003) reached a similar place. So the honest sentence is: yes, there is a measurable effect; it is small; you may well be noticing it; and it is almost certainly smaller than the alternative.

That sentence is very different from "there is no evidence lithium affects memory," which is what people are told, and which is false.

14.4 What Nineteen Years Looks Like

The following account is a composite, with details changed for anonymity.

Xael was 45. Lithium since 26. Two admissions before it, none since, which is the sort of outcome that gets written up as a success and which is a success.

What he wanted to talk about, when he finally raised it, was not a side effect. He had a mild tremor he had stopped noticing. His thyroid was fine. His eGFR was 71 and had been flat for six years. On every measure the clinic tracked, he was a model of what this drug can do.

What he said was that he could not remember what he was like. He had been 26 when he started and he was 45 now, and the whole of his adult character had been formed while medicated, and he had no access to the counterfactual. He did not think the lithium had taken anything. He thought he had no way of knowing whether it had, and that the not-knowing had been quietly present for nineteen years and he had never said it out loud because it sounded, he thought, like the beginning of an argument for stopping.

It was not that. He had no intention of stopping. He was quite clear about that and he had been for years.

His psychiatrist did the thing that was available, which was to say that the question was reasonable, that it had no answer, and that a fair number of people carry it. That was all. There was no intervention. Xael describes the appointment as one of the more useful ones he has had, which tells you something about the bar.

The grief here has no name and no code. It is not depression and it does not respond to a dose change. It is the loss of a version of yourself that never existed, and you cannot mourn it properly because you cannot prove it was there. It is real, it is common, and there is nothing in this book or any other that fixes it. What helps, apparently, is being allowed to say it in a room without anyone reaching for a prescription pad.

> **Teaching Point:** *Excellent outcomes on every measured parameter are compatible with a significant unaddressed cost.*
>
> **Teaching Point:** *Patients withhold this specific complaint because they correctly predict it will be heard as ambivalence about the drug.*

14.5 Where the Decades Bite Hardest

The following is a composite case; identifying details have been changed.

Background Yael, 74, on lithium since her mid-forties. Bipolar I. No episodes in twenty-two years. Living alone. Also taking a blood pressure tablet, a statin, and a tablet for reflux.

Presentation Her daughter brought her in because she had become vague and had fallen twice. The daughter thought it was the beginning of dementia and had come to ask about that.

Analysis Three things had happened at once, none of them individually dramatic. Her renal function had declined gradually with age, so the dose she had taken since 1997 was delivering a higher level than it used to. An ACE inhibitor had been added four years earlier. And she had been eating less, as older people living alone often do, which had reduced her salt intake.

Her level was 1.2 mmol/L on a dose that had not changed in twenty-six years. Not toxic by the usual threshold. And Chapter 8.0 made the point that matters here: the number is not the state. In a 74-year-old with months of slow accumulation, 1.2 was doing what 1.7 would do in her daughter.

The dementia question was not unreasonable. It was just fourth in the queue behind three explanations nobody had checked.

Intervention The lithium dose was reduced by a third. The ACE inhibitor was reviewed and kept, with monitoring. Monitoring was moved to three-monthly, which is what should have happened when she turned 65 and did not, because nothing happens when a person turns 65.

Outcome The vagueness improved substantially over six weeks. She did not fall again in the following year. Some of the cognitive change did not reverse, and whether that residue was lithium, age, or something else beginning is not knowable and her family has had to live with that.

> **Teaching Point:** *A dose that has not changed in twenty-six years is not a stable dose. The person changed.*
>
> **Teaching Point:** *Every sign of lithium excess in an older adult has a more available explanation, and dementia is now at the top of that list rather than the bottom.*
>
> **Teaching Point:** *Monitoring intervals should track age. No mechanism exists to make that happen.*

14.6 The Larger Picture

Xael has filled the organizer nearly a thousand times and does not resent it. Yael took the same dose for twenty-six years and it very nearly cost her her independence, not because anyone was careless but because the arrangement was designed for a woman of 48 and nobody redesigned it for a woman of 74.

Both of those are what success looks like in this field. That is not a criticism. Twenty-two years without an episode is an extraordinary outcome and the drug delivered it. But notice what both stories have in common, which is that the failures were not pharmacological. Nobody prescribed wrongly. What failed was that the treatment was configured once, at a moment, for a person who then went on living for decades, and no part of the system is built to notice the difference between a 26-year-old and the same man at 45, or a 48-year-old and the same woman at 74.

So the question this chapter leaves you with is not whether to take the drug. You have probably settled that, and the evidence in Chapter 1.0 says you should be slow to unsettle it.

The question is this. Your regimen was set up for the person you were when it was set up. How long ago was that, and in what specific ways are you no longer that person? Not your mood. Your kidney, your age, your salt, your other tablets, your job, your rota, the number of people who would notice if you stopped answering the phone. Every one of those has moved since somebody last looked, and the treatment has not moved with them, and there is no appointment at which anyone will ask.

Which leaves one thing left to examine, and it is the one everybody reading this has thought about at three in the morning at least once. Whether to keep doing it at all.

Chapter 15.0: Continuing Switching Stopping

If you have been well for eleven years, what exactly is the evidence that you still need the drug? The question sounds like a trap and it is not. It is the question Kestrel asked in Chapter 1.0 and did not get a straight answer to, and it is the question every person reading this has asked at some point, usually alone, usually at night. The standard reply is that you are well because of the drug, which is circular, and everybody in the room knows it is circular, and the patient concludes that nobody has thought about it properly. The remarkable thing is that there is a real answer. It is not the reassuring one. It has been in the literature since 1991 and it almost never gets said out loud.

15.1 Four Different Conversations Wearing One Name

"I want to come off my medication" is not one sentence. It is four, and they have almost nothing in common except the words.

The intolerable side effect. Cypress in Chapter 11.0. The drug works and the price is one the person is no longer willing to pay. This is a negotiation about the price, and it usually has answers: a different agent, a mechanism identified, a dose reduced.

The medical reason. Wren and Ellis in Chapter 9.0. Kidney function, or a pregnancy, or an interaction with something else that has become necessary. This is an arithmetic problem with two columns.

The doubt about need. Kestrel. The person is well, has been well for years, and wants to know why they are still doing this.

This is an epistemic problem and it has the answer described below.

The illness talking. The person is becoming unwell, and the wish to stop is a symptom rather than a position. This is the one clinicians are most alert to and it is the least common of the four, and the fact that it is the default assumption is why the other three get handled so badly.

Almost every bad conversation about stopping comes from treating one of the first three as though it were the fourth. If you have ever raised this and watched someone's face change, you have seen that misclassification happen in real time.

15.2 The Case That Stopping Is Genuinely Dangerous

Suppes and colleagues (1991) looked at what happens after lithium is discontinued in bipolar disorder. The recurrence rates were high and, more importantly, the timing was not random. Risk concentrated heavily in the first several months after stopping, far in excess of the person's own pre-treatment episode rate.

That last point is the one that matters and it is what makes this more than "the illness comes back." Their own natural history, before they ever took lithium, would not have predicted that many episodes in that window. Something about the stopping itself appeared to generate risk.

Then Faedda and colleagues (1993) found the thing that should be in every discharge letter and is in almost none. Outcome after rapid discontinuation was substantially worse than after gradual discontinuation. Baldessarini and colleagues (1996) confirmed and quantified it: tapering lithium over a matter of weeks rather than days made a large difference to how long people stayed well.

Read that as a patient rather than a researcher. It means the most dangerous version of stopping lithium is the one you do yourself, over a weekend, because you have had enough. Cypress did that in Chapter 11.0. It also means that if you are determined to stop, the single most valuable thing your prescriber can give you is not an argument. It is a taper.

Tondo and colleagues (1998) added the part that gives this chapter its weight: suicidal behavior rises after lithium discontinuation, and the effect is not fully explained by the mood episodes.

Then there is the most contested claim in this area. Post and colleagues (1992) reported preliminary observations of what they called discontinuation-induced refractoriness: the suggestion that some patients who stop lithium and then restart it do not respond as well as they did before. If true, that would change everything, because it would mean stopping carries a risk of permanently losing your best treatment.

15.3 The Case That This Is Overstated

Coryell and colleagues (1998) went looking for refractoriness in a prospective sample and did not find it. Their conclusion was that lithium's effectiveness after discontinuation and restarting was not meaningfully diminished.

That matters enormously and it is not widely known. The refractoriness claim frightens people badly and it is based on a small preliminary report that the best available prospective data did not replicate. I think the honest position is that it may happen in some people and that it is not the general rule, and that presenting it as established, which some clinicians do, is using a weak finding as a compliance tool.

The discontinuation studies have a second problem, and it is real. Most of them are observational and most of them are studying people who stopped, which is not a random group. People stop when they are unwell, or when their life is destabilizing, or when they have decided the drug is not helping. Comparing them to people who continued is comparing two populations that already differed. Some of the excess relapse is confounding by indication, and nobody can say how much.

Third, all of it is about lithium. The discontinuation literature for lamotrigine, valproate, and carbamazepine is thin by comparison, and applying the lithium rebound findings to a person coming off lamotrigine is an extrapolation nobody has earned.

And fourth, the base rate is not zero. Some people stop and stay well. They exist, they are not rare, and they are systematically invisible to psychiatry, because a person who stops their lithium and is fine for fifteen years never comes back to tell anyone.

15.4 What the Evidence Supports and Where It Stops

Three findings are solid enough to act on.

Rapid discontinuation is worse than gradual. This is the strongest practical finding in the whole area and it is actionable regardless of which side of the debate you are on. Weeks, not days. Months is better.

The risk is front-loaded. The first several months after stopping carry most of it. That means a stopping plan needs its intensity at the beginning, which is exactly the opposite of how most of them are run, where the appointments taper alongside the drug.

And the answer to Kestrel's question exists. It is this: your eleven well years are not evidence that you no longer need the drug, and they are not evidence that you do. They are uninformative, because both hypotheses predict them. What is informative is what happened the last time the drug was absent, and what your history looked like before treatment started. That is a real answer to a question she was told was unanswerable. It is not reassuring and it is not circular.

Two things remain genuinely open.

Whether refractoriness is real. Post says maybe, Coryell says no, the sample sizes are what they are, and this will not be settled by argument.

And whether any of this generalizes past lithium. Almost certainly not in the same form, and nobody has done the work.

15.5 Three People Who Decided

The following are composite cases.

Case A Zennor, whose twenty-two months of untreated hypothyroidism opened Chapter 10.0, decided to stop lithium at 44. Her reasoning was that the drug had, in her experience, been accompanied by two years of being ignored, and she no longer trusted the arrangement. That is not a pharmacological reason and it was the actual reason, and it was not the reason recorded in her notes, which said "declines maintenance treatment."

She tapered over five months, which she insisted on and her psychiatrist agreed to. She had a depressive episode at fourteen months, treated as an outpatient. She restarted lithium at sixteen months and it worked as well as it had before. She describes the whole thing as necessary rather than as a mistake.

Case B Ellis, from Chapter 9.0, came off lithium over nine months for his kidney, moved to lamotrigine, and has had one significant depressive episode in the years since.

The two decisions look similar and are not. Ellis was making an arithmetic judgment about an organ, with a bipolar II history and no suicide attempts, and he was moving to another drug rather than to nothing. Zennor was making a judgment about a relationship with a service, with no replacement agent, and she was accepting a relapse risk in exchange for something she could not articulate on a form.

The instructive thing is that both were handled well, and the handling was identical in one respect that mattered more than anything else: both got a taper measured in months rather than a taper measured in whether the clinician approved.

The following account is a composite, with details changed for anonymity.

Kestrel stayed on it. That was where Chapter 1.0 left her: eleven years in, resentful, taking it anyway.

What happened afterward is worth recording because it complicates the tidy version. At fourteen years she asked again. This time she got the answer in 15.4, which is that her well years were uninformative and the informative thing was 2013, the year she stopped for four months in her twenties and ended up in hospital.

She had not forgotten 2013. She had simply never had it placed next to the question. For fourteen years the conversation had been about maintenance treatment in general, and she had been arguing about a principle, and the actual evidence relevant to her was one event in her own history that nobody had brought into the room.

She is still on it. She is still not happy about it. The difference, she says, is that she is now doing it for a reason rather than because someone told her to, and she is aware that this sounds like a small thing and that it took fourteen years.

> **Teaching Point:** *The reason a patient gives for stopping is frequently not the reason recorded, and the recorded one is usually the one the service can act on.*

> **Teaching Point:** *The evidence most relevant to an individual's maintenance decision is usually a specific event in their own history, not a trial.*

15.6 Returning to the Start

Settled:

Stopping lithium abruptly is worse than stopping it slowly, and this is the finding that should be printed on the box. Risk after discontinuation is front-loaded into the first several months. The antisuicidal signal from Chapter 1.0 disappears when the drug does. And nothing here applies straightforwardly to the other three drugs, because nobody has studied them properly.

Contested:

Whether stopping and restarting costs you the drug's future effectiveness. Whether the excess relapse after discontinuation is a rebound phenomenon or confounding by the reasons people stop. And whether the whole discontinuation literature, built largely on people who stopped in the 1980s and 1990s, describes what would happen to a person who tapered slowly, with a replacement agent, under supervision, in 2026.

What this leaves you with is not permission and it is not prohibition.

This book opened by claiming that lithium is first-line because on the two things that matter most over a lifetime, preventing mania and reducing death, nothing has beaten it. Fourteen chapters later that claim still stands and it has acquired a considerable amount of qualification: it is weak against depression, it damages thyroid and parathyroid function, it puts on weight through five separate mechanisms, it becomes dangerous in a heatwave, and it may or may not be doing something slow to your kidney that stopping may or may not reverse.

All of that is true at once. None of it makes the opening claim false. What it does is make the claim conditional, and the condition is the thing this whole book has been about, which is that the risk-benefit ratio only stays favorable if somebody is paying attention.

Kestrel took fourteen years to get a straight answer to a reasonable question. That is the failure this book was written against. Not bad drugs, and not bad doctors. A question asked in year eleven and answered in year fourteen, and the answer having been available in the literature since 1991, and sitting in her own notes since 2013.

So the last thing to say is the first thing. Ask the question. Ask it out loud, ask it of someone who will answer it rather than manage it, and if the answer is circular, say so, because it means they have not looked at your history and the history is where your answer is.

Conclusion: The Prescription Is a Conversation

You now know more about these four drugs than most of the people who will ever prescribe them to you.

That is not a compliment and it is not rhetoric. It is an observation about how medical knowledge is distributed. Your psychiatrist knows an enormous amount about bipolar disorder and holds perhaps forty minutes a year of information about you. A general practitioner writing your repeat prescription has ten minutes and a screen. A pharmacist has your interaction list and not your history. None of them has read fifteen chapters about the specific four drugs you take, because none of them has the time, and none of them needs to, because none of them is taking them.

You have. That asymmetry is the whole of what this book was trying to build.

What Is Negotiable and What Is Not

Almost everything in your treatment is negotiable. The agent. The dose. The timing. Whether the antipsychotic added in 2018 is still earning its place. Whether the sertraline that predates your diagnosis has ever been reviewed against it. Whether your monitoring interval, set when you were 48, is right now that you are 71. Whether you are prepared to keep paying for a drug in weight when a mechanism was never identified. All of that is a conversation, and it is a conversation you are entitled to open.

The physiology is not negotiable. Lithium will impersonate salt in your kidney whatever either of you thinks about it. Lamotrigine's rash window will run from week two to week eight regardless of how much you want to reach the dose faster. Carbamazepine will double its own clearance in the first month whether or not anyone explained that to you. Valproate's neurodevelopmental risk does not care how much the drug has helped you.

The line between those two things is where useful conversations happen. Everything above it is yours to argue about. Everything below it is a fact you build the argument on.

What This Book Could Not Do

Medication is one part of this and I have written as though it were the whole, because that was the brief and the alternative was a worse book. But a person who has read fifteen chapters about pharmacology and nothing about sleep, or routine, or the specific ways relationships absorb this illness, has an incomplete picture and should know it.

The other honest limit is time. Chapter 4.0 has dates in it for a reason. The regulatory position on valproate moved three times in fourteen months: the paternal advice arrived in September 2024, was revised in February 2025, and the patient materials were rewritten again in June 2025. Chapter 9.0's kidney argument was already unsettled by the time this was written, with two studies months apart pointing opposite ways on whether stopping lithium helps the kidney at all. If you are reading this some years after it was written, the pharmacology has not moved and the rules may have, and the way to tell is to check the date on the chapter against the date on your calendar.

The Last Thing

Keep this book. Write in it. The appendices are designed to be defaced.

And when you next sit down in front of someone with a prescription pad, remember what the whole of this was for. Not so you can correct them. Not so you can arrive with a printout and an argument, which is a way of guaranteeing that the ten minutes goes badly.

So that when they say your level is fine, you know that they have told you something true about a number and nothing at all about you, and you know which question to ask next.

That is the difference between a prescription and a conversation. It has taken this entire book to get to it and it fits in a sentence: the drug is theirs to prescribe, and the decade is yours to live, and only one of you is in the room for both.

Appendix A: Master Medication Log

Fill this in once, then update it whenever anything changes. Take it to every appointment. Chapter 6.0 explains why this single sheet is worth more than nine years of notes.

Medication	Dose	Times per day	Start date	What it is for	Who started it

Drugs I have taken before and stopped:

Medication	Dates	Why it stopped (side effect or did not work)

Chapter 4.0 makes a point that belongs on this page. Stopping a drug because you could not tolerate it is a different fact from stopping it because it did not work, and the difference constrains what your prescriber can offer you next. Record which it was.

Allergies and previous drug reactions:

Drugs I cannot take, and why:

Appendix B: Blood Monitoring Log

The twelve hour rule. *A lithium level is only meaningful if the blood was taken approximately twelve hours after your last dose. Write the time of your last dose on the request form every single time. The form has no box for it. Use the margin.*

Date	Time of last dose	Time of blood draw	Lithium level	TSH	Creatinine	eGFR	Calcium	Weight

For valproate: full blood count, liver function tests. **For carbamazepine:** full blood count, liver function tests, sodium. **For lamotrigine:** no routine bloods required. In pregnancy, levels are monitored.

Date	FBC	LFT	Sodium	Other

My creatinine before I started lithium was: ___________
(Chapter 9.0 explains why this number predicts your risk and why it is worth finding.)

Appendix C: eGFR Trend Chart

One eGFR tells you almost nothing. Five over six years tell you a great deal. Nobody else is plotting this. Plot it.

eGFR	Year 1	Year 2	Year 3	Year 4	Year 5	Year 6	Year 7	Year 8
100 or above								
90 to 99								
80 to 89								
70 to 79								
60 to 69								
50 to 59								
40 to 49								
30 to 39								
Below 30								

Put a mark in the cell that matches each year's value. What you are looking for is not a number. It is a slope.

Things that affect this slope other than lithium (from Chapter 9.0):

- Blood pressure. Often doing more damage than the lithium and easier to fix.

- Age. Everyone's eGFR declines with age.
- Diabetes.
- Episodes of toxicity.

Appendix D: Lamotrigine Titration Calendar and Rash Red Flags

The slow climb is not caution. It is the intervention. Chapter 3.0 explains why.

Standard adult titration (lamotrigine alone, no valproate):

Weeks	Dose
1 and 2	25 mg daily
3 and 4	50 mg daily
5	100 mg daily
6	200 mg daily
7 onward	Maintenance, usually 200 mg daily

If you are also taking valproate: the doses are roughly halved and the climb is slower. Valproate doubles your lamotrigine level. If valproate was added and your lamotrigine dose did not change, ask why.

If you are also taking carbamazepine: doses are typically higher, because carbamazepine speeds up lamotrigine clearance.

> ***If you miss five or more days****, do not restart at your usual dose. You start the climb again from the beginning. Doubling up to catch up is more dangerous than the gap.*

Rash red flags: weeks 2 to 8

Stop the drug and be seen the same day if a rash comes with any of these:

- **Fever** (the one people misread as evidence of a virus)
- Sores or blisters in the mouth, eyes, throat, or genitals

- Blistering or peeling anywhere
- Skin that hurts rather than itches
- Swollen glands
- Feeling ill all over, the way flu feels ill
- Rash on the face and upper trunk

If none of those are present: photograph it with the date, phone rather than panic. On the mood disorder trial figures, benign rashes outnumber serious ones by roughly 60 to one. The 0.3% in the boxed warning is the epilepsy figure, not yours.

The window reopens if valproate is added at any point.

Appendix E: Pregnancy Comparison, Four Drugs

Absolute numbers, not relative risk. Chapter 12.0 sets these out in full and explains why the second column is the one that never appears in the room.

Drug	Major malformation risk	Neurodevelopmental risk	Notes
Valproate	Approx. 3 to 5% neural tube defects; approx. 1 in 9 overall major malformation (MHRA figure); highest of eight antiepileptics (EURAP)	Approx. 30 to 40% (3 to 4 in 10) of exposed children	Dose-related. Also lower birth weight for gestational age (MHRA, June 2025). Restricted: see Appendix L.
Carbamazepine	Approx. 1% neural tube defects	Signal present but far below valproate	Also renders hormonal contraception unreliable
Lithium	Cardiac malformation 2.41 per 100 exposed vs 1.15 per 100 unexposed (adj. RR 1.65, 95% CI 1.02 to 2.68). RVOTO defects 0.60 per 100 vs 0.18 per	No comparable signal	The historical 400-fold Ebstein's figure came from a voluntary register and was wrong. Clearance rises in pregnancy.

Drug	Major malformation risk	Neurodevelopmental risk	Notes
	100 (adj. RR 2.66, 95% CI 1.00 to 7.06)		
Lamotrigine	Lowest of the group (EURAP); 1.39 per 100 cardiac in the Patorno comparison	No autism signal found (Hernández-Díaz et al., 2024)	Clearance rises substantially in pregnancy; dose must climb, then fall after delivery

The other column

	Risk
Recurrence in pregnancy after **discontinuing** a mood stabiliser	**85.5%** (Viguera et al., 2007a)
Recurrence in pregnancy while **continuing**	**37%**
Recurrence across the whole cohort, both groups	71%
Proportion of pregnancy spent unwell, discontinued vs continued	over 40% vs 8.8%
Postpartum relapse, bipolar disorder	**37%** (Wesseloo et al., 2016)
Postpartum relapse, **medication free** in pregnancy	**66%**
Postpartum relapse, **on prophylaxis**	**23%**
Severe postpartum episode, bipolar disorder	17%
Severe postpartum episode, prior postpartum psychosis	29%

Question to take to the appointment: what is my risk of relapse if I stop, what is it if I continue, and can I see both numbers on the same page before I decide?

Appendix F: Early Warning Agreement

Complete this on a good day, with the person who would notice. Chapter 13.0 explains why this fifteen minutes is worth more than a year of appointments.

The two or three signs that matter most for me (be specific; sleep is usually first):

1. ____ 2. ____ 3. ____

The sentence you are allowed to say to me (make it about an observation, not about me):

____

What happens when you say it:

I will ______________________________________ within ________ hours. And that is all that happens. No argument, no consequence, no discussion of whether you were right.

The override. The specific circumstance in which you act regardless of what I say at the time:

____

(For lithium, this is usually: unsteady, slurring, or a tremor that has changed character.)

Signed: ______________________ **Date:** ____________

Signed: ______________________ **Date:** ____________

Review this every year. The signs change.

Appendix G: Appointment Agenda

Ten minutes. Take one thing, not five. Fill this in before you go.

The one thing I want from this appointment:

____

____

My last blood results and their dates:

Test	Value	Date
Lithium level		
TSH		
eGFR		
Calcium		

Anything that has changed since last time (new tablets from anyone, including a pharmacy shelf; illness; weight; sleep; alcohol; work):

____

____

Questions worth asking, if they fit:

- Which of my four boxes were checked this time, and which were not?
- My calcium has not been checked since __________. Should it be?
- Is my monitoring interval still right for my age?
- Drug __________ has been in my regimen since __________ and I do not know what problem it is solving. What is it for?

- What would have to be true for us to review it?

Appendix H: Continue, Switch, or Stop Ledger

Chapter 15.0 argues that "I want to come off my medication" is four different conversations. Work out which one you are having before you have it.

Which is this?

- The price is too high (a side effect I am no longer willing to pay for)
- There is a medical reason (kidney, pregnancy, an interaction)
- I doubt I still need it
- Something else

If the price is too high: which mechanism? (Chapter 11.0 for weight; Chapter 10.0 for tiredness.) Has anyone identified it, or was I given advice?

If I doubt I still need it: the informative question is not how long I have been well. It is:

- What happened the last time I was without this drug? Date: __________ Outcome: __________
- What did my history look like before treatment? __________

If we are going ahead:

Taper over	________ months (weeks is worse than months; days is worst of all)
Replacement agent	_________ or none

Appointments concentrated in the first	________ months (the risk is front-loaded)
Who is watching (Appendix F)	__________
What we do if there is a wobble	Pause and hold, or restore? (A wobble is information about the rate, not proof of necessity.)

Appendix I: Sick Day and Hot Weather Card

Cut this out. Put it somewhere it will be found by someone who is not well.

I take lithium.

My level rises when I am dry. *Vomiting, diarrhea, fever, heat, heavy sweating, hard exercise, drinking less, eating less salt. Any of these lasting more than about 24 hours is a lithium event.*

What to do:

1. Contact my prescriber or an out-of-hours service.

2. Say the word **lithium** *in the first sentence.*

3. Ask for a level.

4. Take fluids with some salt in them, not plain water alone.

5. Do not decide to skip doses on my own.

If I am becoming unsteady, drowsy, or my tremor has changed: *that is an emergency department, today. Say lithium first.*

At every pharmacy counter, in every country, before anything is handed over:

"I take lithium. Is this safe with lithium?"

Not "I take medication for my mental health."

Raise my level: *ibuprofen and other anti-inflammatories, ACE inhibitors and sartans, thiazide diuretics, dehydration, low salt.*

Safe for pain: *paracetamol (acetaminophen).*

Appendix J: Emergency Signs, All Four Drugs

Lithium: toxicity

Early: tremor changes character (coarser, slower, larger). Nausea. Loose stools. Feeling unwell without a location. **Middle:** unsteadiness, walking as though drunk. Slurred speech. Drowsiness that is not tiredness. Muscle twitching. **Act here.** **Late:** confusion, seizures, reduced consciousness.

The number is not the state. Chronic toxicity is dangerous at a lower level than an overdose is. Do not wait for a level.

Lamotrigine: hypersensitivity

Rash with fever, mucosal involvement (mouth, eyes, throat, genitals), blistering, or feeling ill all over. Weeks 2 to 8 mainly, and again if valproate is added. **Stop and be seen today.**

Carbamazepine

Blood: fever, sore throat, mouth ulcers, unexplained bruising. Needs a full blood count today, not antibiotics. **Sodium:** confusion, unsteadiness, a fall, headache, vagueness. Needs a sodium.

Valproate

Pancreas: persistent vomiting with abdominal pain radiating to the back. **Liver:** jaundice, dark urine, unusual bruising, profound lethargy. More common in the first six months.

The pattern in all four: the emergency presents as something ordinary, the ordinary explanation is more likely, and the thing that distinguishes them is a test that will not be ordered unless somebody names the drug.

Appendix K: Brand Names by Country

Brands are not interchangeable, particularly for lithium. A substitution is a dose change and requires a level check.

Drug	UK	US	Australia	Elsewhere in Europe
Lithium carbonate	Priadel, Camcolit, Liskonum	Lithobid, Eskalith (discontinued in some markets)	Lithicarb, Quilonum SR	Quilonorm, Hypnorex, Carbolithium
Lithium citrate	Priadel liquid, Li-Liquid	Various generic		
Valproate / divalproex	Epilim, Depakote, Episenta, Convulex	Depakote, Depakene, Stavzor	Epilim, Valpro	Depakine, Orfiril, Ergenyl
Lamotrigine	Lamictal	Lamictal	Lamictal, Lamotrust	Lamictal, Lamotrigin
Carbamazepine	Tegretol, Carbagen	Tegretol, Carbatrol, Equetro	Tegretol, Teril	Tegretol, Timonil

Note that lithium carbonate and lithium citrate contain different amounts of lithium and are not swapped like for like. Prescriptions are written by brand for this reason. If yours has quietly changed, your next level is not comparable to your last one.

Appendix L: Valproate Pathways

Three pathways. Find yours. Dates matter because this has moved three times in fourteen months. Chapter 4.0 has the full account.

Pathway 1: Anyone under 55 being started on valproate (from 31 January 2024)

Male or female. Valproate must not be started unless:

- **Two specialists independently** consider and document that there is no other effective or tolerated treatment, **or**
- that the reproductive risks do not apply.

Pathway 2: Woman or girl able to become pregnant, already taking valproate

- Pregnancy Prevention Programme
- Highly effective contraception
- Annual Risk Acknowledgement Form
- Annual specialist review. Two specialists sign off continuation at the first annual review under the revised process; one specialist at subsequent reviews, in consultation with you.

> ***The exemption almost nobody is told about:*** *the framework permits continuation where there are compelling reasons that the reproductive risks do not apply. If pregnancy is not a possibility for you, those are the words. They are in the framework and they are yours to use.*

Pathway 3: Man under 55, already taking valproate (as revised February 2025)

- Dual specialist review **no longer required** (changed 13 February 2025)
- You and your partner are advised to use effective contraception during treatment and for three months after stopping (September 2024 advice)
- At each review you will be asked whether you plan to start a family within the next year. If so, referral to discuss alternatives.

> ***The honest note.*** *The paternal measures rest on one retrospective observational study. An evidence review found no clear evidence of an adverse impact of paternal antiseizure medication use on offspring outcomes. The regulatory position was revised within six months. You are entitled to know that the evidence here is thin and contested. The maternal evidence is neither.*

Updated June 2025: the safety and educational materials were revised again, without changing the rules above. The revision added a risk of lower birth weight for gestational age after exposure in pregnancy.

Check the date. This is the fastest-moving content in this book. As of this edition the last substantive change was February 2025 and the last materials update was June 2025.

Appendix M: Glossary

Ataxia. Unsteady, uncoordinated movement. Walking as though drunk. A middle-stage sign of lithium toxicity.

Autoinduction. A drug increasing the enzymes that clear it, so the same dose delivers less over time. Carbamazepine does this over roughly three to five weeks.

CYP3A4. A liver enzyme that clears a very large proportion of medications. Carbamazepine turns it up, which is why it weakens so many other drugs, including hormonal contraception.

eGFR. Estimated glomerular filtration rate. A calculated measure of kidney function. The trend matters; a single value does not.

Enzyme induction. Speeding up the liver's clearance of drugs. Carbamazepine is a strong inducer.

Enzyme inhibition. Slowing it down. Valproate inhibits the enzyme that clears lamotrigine, roughly doubling lamotrigine levels.

Hypercalcemia. Raised blood calcium. Associated with long-term lithium via the parathyroid glands. Symptoms: tiredness, low mood, constipation, thirst, poor concentration, all of which have three other explanations.

Hyponatremia. Low blood sodium. Common on carbamazepine. Presents as vagueness, unsteadiness, falls, or headache.

Hypothyroidism. Underactive thyroid. Affects roughly 6 to 20% of long-term lithium patients, more in women. Presents identically to depression except for cold intolerance.

Narrow therapeutic index. A small gap between the dose that works and the dose that harms. Lithium's is roughly a factor of two and a half. This is why the blood tests exist.

Nephrogenic diabetes insipidus. The kidney losing its ability to concentrate urine. Produces thirst and large volumes of dilute urine. Common on lithium, largely reversible, and not the same thing as kidney damage. Nothing to do with diabetes mellitus.

Neural tube defect. A malformation of the developing spine or brain, including spina bifida. Valproate approx. 3 to 5%; carbamazepine approx. 1%.

Prodrome. The early signs of an episode beginning, before it is established. Sleep usually goes first.

Stevens-Johnson syndrome / toxic epidermal necrolysis. Severe immune skin reactions in which the epidermis detaches. Treated in burns units. The reason lamotrigine is titrated slowly.

Teratogen. A substance that causes malformation in a developing fetus.

Titration. Stepping a dose up gradually. For lamotrigine, the titration is not caution. It is the safety mechanism itself.

Trough level. A blood level taken at the low point of the dosing cycle. For lithium, approximately twelve hours after the last dose. Every reference range assumes this.

TSH. Thyroid stimulating hormone. The pituitary shouting at the thyroid. Rises before thyroid hormone levels fall far enough to look abnormal, which is why it is the early warning number.

Appendix N: Where to Look Next

Regulatory and guideline sources

- Medicines and Healthcare products Regulatory Agency (MHRA) Drug Safety Update. The primary source for the valproate position and the one that changes. Check the date on anything you read about valproate, including Appendix L of this book.
- National Institute for Health and Care Excellence, Clinical Guideline CG185, *Bipolar disorder: assessment and management*. The source of the six-monthly monitoring schedule.
- National Institute for Health and Care Excellence, Clinical Guideline CG192, *Antenatal and postnatal mental health.*
- Canadian Network for Mood and Anxiety Treatments and International Society for Bipolar Disorders (CANMAT/ISBD) guidelines. The most detailed international treatment guidance.
- British Association for Psychopharmacology bipolar guidelines.

Medicines information

- Electronic Medicines Compendium (UK) and DailyMed (US). The full Summary of Product Characteristics, which is the long version of the leaflet in your box and contains considerably more than the leaflet does.
- LactMed, for breastfeeding and medication. The best free source on this and better than most clinicians' recollection.
- UK Teratology Information Service, for pregnancy exposures.

Patient organizations

- Bipolar UK.
- Depression and Bipolar Support Alliance (US).
- Action on Postpartum Psychosis, for anything in the territory of Chapter 12.0.
- The Independent Medicines and Medical Devices Safety Review (the Cumberlege review, *First Do No Harm*, 2020), for the valproate history in Chapter 4.0 and for what it says about what happens when patients report harm and are not believed.

A note on searching

If you search for "lithium kidney" you will find the 1970s and 1980s literature first, because it is older and more cited and more frightening. Chapter 9.0 exists because of that. Add a year filter. The picture from 2015 onward is a different picture, and it is still not settled, and the unsettledness is the honest finding rather than a gap in your search.

References

Adityanjee, Munshi, K. R., & Thampy, A. (2005). The syndrome of irreversible lithium-effectuated neurotoxicity. *Clinical Neuropharmacology*, *28*(1), 38-49. https://doi.org/10.1097/01.wnf.0000150871.52253.b7

Aiff, H., Attman, P. O., Aurell, M., Bendz, H., Schön, S., & Svedlund, J. (2014). The impact of modern treatment principles may have eliminated lithium-induced renal failure. *Journal of Psychopharmacology*, *28*(2), 151-154. https://doi.org/10.1177/0269881113516202

Aiff, H., Attman, P. O., Aurell, M., Bendz, H., Ramsauer, B., Schön, S., & Svedlund, J. (2015). Effects of 10 to 30 years of lithium treatment on kidney function. *Journal of Psychopharmacology*, *29*(5), 608-614. https://doi.org/10.1177/0269881115573808

Albert, U., De Cori, D., Aguglia, A., Barbaro, F., Bogetto, F., & Maina, G. (2013). Lithium-associated hyperparathyroidism and hypercalcaemia: A case-control cross-sectional study. *Journal of Affective Disorders*, *151*(2), 786-790. https://doi.org/10.1016/j.jad.2013.06.046

Alda, M. (2015). Lithium in the treatment of bipolar disorder: Pharmacology and pharmacogenetics. *Molecular Psychiatry*, *20*(6), 661-670. https://doi.org/10.1038/mp.2015.4

Amdisen, A. (1977). Serum level monitoring and clinical pharmacokinetics of lithium. *Clinical Pharmacokinetics*, *2*(2), 73-92. https://doi.org/10.2165/00003088-197702020-00001

American Psychiatric Association. (2022). *Diagnostic and statistical manual of mental disorders* (5th ed., text rev.).

American Psychiatric Association Publishing. https://doi.org/10.1176/appi.books.9780890425787

Anderson, G. D. (1998). A mechanistic approach to antiepileptic drug interactions. *Annals of Pharmacotherapy*, *32*(5), 554-563. https://doi.org/10.1345/aph.17332

Attri, J. P., Bala, N., & Chatrath, V. (2012). Psychiatric patient and anaesthesia. *Indian Journal of Anaesthesia*, *56*(1), 8-13. https://doi.org/10.4103/0019-5049.93337

Baird-Gunning, J., Lea-Henry, T., Hoegberg, L. C. G., Gosselin, S., & Roberts, D. M. (2017). Lithium poisoning. *Journal of Intensive Care Medicine*, *32*(4), 249-263. https://doi.org/10.1177/0885066616651582

BALANCE investigators and collaborators. (2010). Lithium plus valproate combination therapy versus monotherapy for relapse prevention in bipolar I disorder (BALANCE): A randomised open-label trial. *The Lancet*, *375*(9712), 385-395. https://doi.org/10.1016/S0140-6736(09)61828-6

Baldessarini, R. J., Tondo, L., Faedda, G. L., Suppes, T. R., Floris, G., & Rudas, N. (1996). Effects of the rate of discontinuing lithium maintenance treatment in bipolar disorders. *Journal of Clinical Psychiatry*, *57*(10), 441-448. https://doi.org/10.4088/jcp.v57n1001

Baldessarini, R. J., Tondo, L., & Viguera, A. C. (1999). Discontinuing lithium maintenance treatment in bipolar disorders: Risks and implications. *Bipolar Disorders*, *1*(1), 17-24. https://doi.org/10.1034/j.1399-5618.1999.10106.x

Baldessarini, R. J., & Tondo, L. (2000). Does lithium treatment still work? Evidence of stable responses over three decades. *Archives of General Psychiatry*, *57*(2), 187-190. https://doi.org/10.1001/archpsyc.57.2.187

Baldessarini, R. J., Tondo, L., Davis, P., Pompili, M., Goodwin, F. K., & Hennen, J. (2006). Decreased risk of suicides and attempts during long-term lithium treatment: A meta-analytic review. *Bipolar Disorders*, *8*(5p2), 625-639. https://doi.org/10.1111/j.1399-5618.2006.00344.x

Baldessarini, R., Henk, H., Sklar, A., Chang, J., & Leahy, L. (2008). Psychotropic medications for patients with bipolar disorder in the United States: Polytherapy and adherence. *Psychiatric Services*, *59*(10), 1175-1183. https://doi.org/10.1176/ps.2008.59.10.1175

Batlle, D. C., von Riotte, A. B., Gaviria, M., & Grupp, M. (1985). Amelioration of polyuria by amiloride in patients receiving long-term lithium therapy. *New England Journal of Medicine*, *312*(7), 408-414. https://doi.org/10.1056/NEJM198502143120705

Bauer, M., & Gitlin, M. (2016). *The essential guide to lithium treatment*. Springer. https://doi.org/10.1007/978-3-319-31214-9

Bendz, H., Schön, S., Attman, P. O., & Aurell, M. (2010). Renal failure occurs in chronic lithium treatment but is uncommon. *Kidney International*, *77*(3), 219-224. https://doi.org/10.1038/ki.2009.433

Berghuis, B., van der Palen, J., de Haan, G. J., Lindhout, D., Koeleman, B. P. C., Sander, J. W., & EpiPGX Consortium. (2017). Carbamazepine- and oxcarbazepine-induced hyponatremia in people with epilepsy. *Epilepsia*, *58*(7), 1227-1233. https://doi.org/10.1111/epi.13777

Bergink, V., Bouvy, P. F., Vervoort, J. S., Koorengevel, K. M., Steegers, E. A., & Kushner, S. A. (2012). Prevention of postpartum psychosis and mania in women at high risk. *American Journal of Psychiatry*, *169*(6), 609-615. https://doi.org/10.1176/appi.ajp.2012.11071047

Berk, M., Berk, L., Dodd, S., Cotton, S., Macneil, C., Daglas, R., Conus, P., Bechdolf, A., Moylan, S., & Malhi, G. S. (2014).

Stage managing bipolar disorder. *Bipolar Disorders*, *16*(5), 471-477. https://doi.org/10.1111/bdi.12099

Bernus, I., Dickinson, R. G., Hooper, W. D., & Eadie, M. J. (1997). The mechanism of the carbamazepine and valproate interaction in humans. *British Journal of Clinical Pharmacology*, *44*(1), 21-27. https://doi.org/10.1046/j.1365-2125.1997.00607.x

Bertilsson, L., Höjer, B., Tybring, G., Osterloh, J., & Rane, A. (1980). Autoinduction of carbamazepine metabolism in children examined by a stable isotope technique. *Clinical Pharmacology and Therapeutics*, *27*(1), 83-88. https://doi.org/10.1038/clpt.1980.13

Bocchetta, A., & Loviselli, A. (2006). Lithium treatment and thyroid abnormalities. *Clinical Practice and Epidemiology in Mental Health*, *2*, 23. https://doi.org/10.1186/1745-0179-2-23

Bocchetta, A., Cocco, F., Velluzzi, F., Del Zompo, M., Mariotti, S., & Loviselli, A. (2007). Fifteen-year follow-up of thyroid function in lithium patients. *Journal of Endocrinological Investigation*, *30*(5), 363-366. https://doi.org/10.1007/BF03346311

Boton, R., Gaviria, M., & Batlle, D. C. (1987). Prevalence, pathogenesis, and treatment of renal dysfunction associated with chronic lithium therapy. *American Journal of Kidney Diseases*, *10*(5), 329-345. https://doi.org/10.1016/s0272-6386(87)80098-7

Bowden, C. L., Brugger, A. M., Swann, A. C., Calabrese, J. R., Janicak, P. G., Petty, F., Dilsaver, S. C., Davis, J. M., Rush, A. J., Small, J. G., Garza-Trevino, E. S., Risch, S. C., Goodnick, P. J., & Morris, D. D. (1994). Efficacy of divalproex vs lithium and placebo in the treatment of mania.

JAMA, *271*(12), 918-924. https://doi.org/10.1001/jama.1994.03510360044034

Bowden, C. L., Calabrese, J. R., Sachs, G., Yatham, L. N., Asghar, S. A., Hompland, M., Montgomery, P., Earl, N., Smoot, T. M., & DeVeaugh-Geiss, J. (2003). A placebo-controlled 18-month trial of lamotrigine and lithium maintenance treatment in recently manic or hypomanic patients with bipolar I disorder. *Archives of General Psychiatry*, *60*(4), 392-400. https://doi.org/10.1001/archpsyc.60.4.392

Bowden, C. L., Calabrese, J. R., Ketter, T. A., Sachs, G. S., White, R. L., & Thompson, T. R. (2006). Impact of lamotrigine and lithium on weight in obese and nonobese patients with bipolar I disorder. *American Journal of Psychiatry*, *163*(7), 1199-1201. https://doi.org/10.1176/ajp.2006.163.7.1199

Bromley, R. L., Mawer, G. E., Briggs, M., Cheyne, C., Clayton-Smith, J., García-Fiñana, M., Kneen, R., Lucas, S. B., Shallcross, R., & Baker, G. A. (2013). The prevalence of neurodevelopmental disorders in children prenatally exposed to antiepileptic drugs. *Journal of Neurology, Neurosurgery and Psychiatry*, *84*(6), 637-643. https://doi.org/10.1136/jnnp-2012-304270

Cade, J. F. J. (1949). Lithium salts in the treatment of psychotic excitement. *Medical Journal of Australia*, *2*(10), 349-352. https://doi.org/10.5694/j.1326-5377.1949.tb36912.x

Calabrese, J. R., Bowden, C. L., Sachs, G. S., Ascher, J. A., Monaghan, E., & Rudd, G. D. (1999). A double-blind placebo-controlled study of lamotrigine monotherapy in outpatients with bipolar I depression. *Journal of Clinical Psychiatry*, *60*(2), 79-88. https://doi.org/10.4088/jcp.v60n0203

Calabrese, J. R., Sullivan, J. R., Bowden, C. L., Suppes, T., Goldberg, J. F., Sachs, G. S., Shelton, M. D., Goodwin, F.

K., Frye, M. A., & Kusumakar, V. (2002). Rash in multicenter trials of lamotrigine in mood disorders: Clinical relevance and management. *Journal of Clinical Psychiatry, 63*(11), 1012-1019. https://doi.org/10.4088/jcp.v63n1110

Ceron-Litvoc, D., Soares, B. G., Geddes, J., Litvoc, J., & de Lima, M. S. (2009). Comparison of carbamazepine and lithium in treatment of bipolar disorder: A systematic review of randomized controlled trials. *Human Psychopharmacology, 24*(1), 19-28. https://doi.org/10.1002/hup.990

Chen, Y., & Silverstone, T. (1990). Lithium and weight gain. *International Clinical Psychopharmacology*, *5*(3), 217-225. https://doi.org/10.1097/00004850-199007000-00005

Chen, P., Lin, J. J., Lu, C. S., Ong, C. T., Hsieh, P. F., Yang, C. C., Tai, C. T., Wu, S. L., Lu, C. H., Hsu, Y. C., Yu, H. Y., Ro, L. S., Lu, C. T., Chu, C. C., Tsai, J. J., Su, Y. H., Lan, S. H., Sung, S. F., Lin, S. Y., … Taiwan SJS Consortium. (2011). Carbamazepine-induced toxic effects and HLA-B*1502 screening in Taiwan.* New England Journal of Medicine, 364*(12), 1126-1133. https://doi.org/10.1056/NEJMoa1009717

Christensen, J., Grønborg, T. K., Sørensen, M. J., Schendel, D., Parner, E. T., Pedersen, L. H., & Vestergaard, M. (2013). Prenatal valproate exposure and risk of autism spectrum disorders and childhood autism. *JAMA*, *309*(16), 1696-1703. https://doi.org/10.1001/jama.2013.2270

Chung, W. H., Hung, S. I., Hong, H. S., Hsih, M. S., Yang, L. C., Ho, H. C., Wu, J. Y., & Chen, Y. T. (2004). Medical genetics: A marker for Stevens-Johnson syndrome. *Nature*, *428*(6982), 486. https://doi.org/10.1038/428486a

Cipriani, A., Hawton, K., Stockton, S., & Geddes, J. R. (2013). Lithium in the prevention of suicide in mood disorders:

Updated systematic review and meta-analysis. *BMJ*, *346*, f3646. https://doi.org/10.1136/bmj.f3646

Clos, S., Rauchhaus, P., Severn, A., Cochrane, L., & Donnan, P. T. (2015). Long-term effect of lithium maintenance therapy on estimated glomerular filtration rate in patients with affective disorders: A population-based cohort study. *The Lancet Psychiatry*, *2*(12), 1075-1083. https://doi.org/10.1016/S2215-0366(15)00316-8

Cohen, L. S., Friedman, J. M., Jefferson, J. W., Johnson, E. M., & Weiner, M. L. (1994). A reevaluation of risk of in utero exposure to lithium. *JAMA*, *271*(2), 146-150. https://doi.org/10.1001/jama.1994.03510260078033

Collins, N., Barnes, T. R. E., Shingleton-Smith, A., Gerrett, D., & Paton, C. (2010). Standards of lithium monitoring in mental health trusts in the UK. *BMC Psychiatry*, *10*, 80. https://doi.org/10.1186/1471-244X-10-80

Colom, F., Vieta, E., Sánchez-Moreno, J., Palomino-Otiniano, R., Reinares, M., Goikolea, J. M., Benabarre, A., & Martínez-Arán, A. (2009). Group psychoeducation for stabilised bipolar disorders: 5-year outcome of a randomised clinical trial. *British Journal of Psychiatry*, *194*(3), 260-265. https://doi.org/10.1192/bjp.bp.107.040485

Coryell, W., Solomon, D., Leon, A. C., Akiskal, H. S., Keller, M. B., Scheftner, W. A., & Mueller, T. (1998). Lithium discontinuation and subsequent effectiveness. *American Journal of Psychiatry*, *155*(7), 895-898. https://doi.org/10.1176/ajp.155.7.895

Crawford, P. (2002). Interactions between antiepileptic drugs and hormonal contraception. *CNS Drugs*, *16*(4), 263-272. https://doi.org/10.2165/00023210-200216040-00005

Cumberlege, J. (2020). *First do no harm: The report of the Independent Medicines and Medical Devices Safety Review*.

Independent Medicines and Medical Devices Safety Review. https://www.iMMDSreview.org.uk

Davis, J., Desmond, M., & Berk, M. (2018). Lithium and nephrotoxicity: A literature review of approaches to clinical management and risk stratification. *BMC Nephrology*, *19*, 305. https://doi.org/10.1186/s12882-018-1101-4

Decker, B. S., Goldfarb, D. S., Dargan, P. I., Friesen, M., Gosselin, S., Hoffman, R. S., Lavergne, V., Nolin, T. D., Ghannoum, M., & EXTRIP Workgroup. (2015). Extracorporeal treatment for lithium poisoning: Systematic review and recommendations from the EXTRIP workgroup. *Clinical Journal of the American Society of Nephrology*, *10*(5), 875-887. https://doi.org/10.2215/CJN.10021014

DiLiberti, J. H., Farndon, P. A., Dennis, N. R., & Curry, C. J. (1984). The fetal valproate syndrome. *American Journal of Medical Genetics*, *19*(3), 473-481. https://doi.org/10.1002/ajmg.1320190308

Duan, Y., Qiu, F., Zhou, J., Liu, S., Zhao, D., & Qiu, C. (2023). Case report: Progressive skin rash and lymphadenopathy associated with lamotrigine and valproic acid combination in a bipolar adolescent. *Frontiers in Pharmacology*, *14*, 1106423. https://doi.org/10.3389/fphar.2023.1106423

Eichelbaum, M., Ekbom, K., Bertilsson, L., Ringberger, V. A., & Rane, A. (1975). Plasma kinetics of carbamazepine and its epoxide metabolite in man after single and multiple doses. *European Journal of Clinical Pharmacology*, *8*(5), 337-341. https://doi.org/10.1007/BF00562658

Faedda, G. L., Tondo, L., Baldessarini, R. J., Suppes, T., & Tohen, M. (1993). Outcome after rapid vs gradual discontinuation of lithium treatment in bipolar disorders. *Archives of General Psychiatry*, *50*(6), 448-455. https://doi.org/10.1001/archpsyc.1993.01820180046005

Fagiolini, A., Frank, E., Houck, P. R., Mallinger, A. G., Swartz, H. A., Buysse, D. J., Ombao, H., & Kupfer, D. J. (2002). Prevalence of obesity and weight change during treatment in patients with bipolar I disorder. *Journal of Clinical Psychiatry*, *63*(6), 528-533. https://doi.org/10.4088/jcp.v63n0611

Ferrell, P. B., & McLeod, H. L. (2008). Carbamazepine, HLA-B*1502 and risk of Stevens-Johnson syndrome and toxic epidermal necrolysis: US FDA recommendations.* Pharmacogenomics, 9*(10), 1543-1546. https://doi.org/10.2217/14622416.9.10.1543

Finley, P. R. (2016). Drug interactions with lithium: An update. *Clinical Pharmacokinetics*, *55*(8), 925-941. https://doi.org/10.1007/s40262-016-0370-y

Fornaro, M., Maritan, E., Ferranti, R., Zaninotto, L., Miola, A., Anastasia, A., Murru, A., Solé, E., Stubbs, B., Carvalho, A. F., Serretti, A., Vieta, E., Fusar-Poli, P., McGuire, P., Young, A. H., Dazzan, P., Vigod, S. N., Correll, C. U., & Solmi, M. (2020). Lithium exposure during pregnancy and the postpartum period: A systematic review and meta-analysis of safety and efficacy outcomes. *American Journal of Psychiatry*, *177*(1), 76-92. https://doi.org/10.1176/appi.ajp.2019.19030228

Fountoulakis, K. N., Yatham, L., Grunze, H., Vieta, E., Young, A., Blier, P., Kasper, S., & Moeller, H. J. (2017). The International College of Neuro-Psychopharmacology (CINP) treatment guidelines for bipolar disorder in adults (CINP-BD-2017), part 2: Review, grading of the evidence, and a precise algorithm. *International Journal of Neuropsychopharmacology*, *20*(2), 121-179. https://doi.org/10.1093/ijnp/pyw100

Fransson, F., Werneke, U., Öhlund, L., Jonsson, P. A., & Ott, M. (2025). Kidney function decline improves after lithium discontinuation. *Journal of Internal Medicine*, *297*(3), 289-299. https://doi.org/10.1111/joim.20054

Frey, N., Bodmer, M., Bircher, A., Jick, S. S., Meier, C. R., & Spoendlin, J. (2017). The risk of Stevens-Johnson syndrome and toxic epidermal necrolysis in new users of antiepileptic drugs. *Epilepsia*, *58*(12), 2178-2185. https://doi.org/10.1111/epi.13925

Frye, M. A., Denicoff, K. D., Bryan, A. L., Smith-Jackson, E. E., Ali, S. O., Luckenbaugh, D., Leverich, G. S., & Post, R. M. (1999). Association between lower serum free T4 and greater mood instability and depression in lithium-maintained bipolar patients. *American Journal of Psychiatry*, *156*(12), 1909-1914. https://doi.org/10.1176/ajp.156.12.1909

Geddes, J. R., Burgess, S., Hawton, K., Jamison, K., & Goodwin, G. M. (2004). Long-term lithium therapy for bipolar disorder: Systematic review and meta-analysis of randomized controlled trials. *American Journal of Psychiatry*, *161*(2), 217-222. https://doi.org/10.1176/appi.ajp.161.2.217

Geddes, J. R., Calabrese, J. R., & Goodwin, G. M. (2009). Lamotrigine for treatment of bipolar depression: Independent meta-analysis and meta-regression of individual patient data from five randomised trials. *British Journal of Psychiatry*, *194*(1), 4-9. https://doi.org/10.1192/bjp.bp.107.048504

Geddes, J. R., & Miklowitz, D. J. (2013). Treatment of bipolar disorder. *The Lancet*, *381*(9878), 1672-1682. https://doi.org/10.1016/S0140-6736(13)60857-0

Gitlin, M. (2016). Lithium side effects and toxicity: Prevalence and management strategies. *International Journal of Bipolar Disorders*, *4*, 27. https://doi.org/10.1186/s40345-016-0068-y

Goldberg, J. F., Perlis, R. H., Ghaemi, S. N., Calabrese, J. R., Bowden, C. L., Wisniewski, S., Miklowitz, D. J., Sachs, G. S., & Thase, M. E. (2007). Adjunctive antidepressant use and symptomatic recovery among bipolar depressed patients with concomitant manic symptoms: Findings from the STEP-BD. *American Journal of Psychiatry*, *164*(9), 1348-1355. https://doi.org/10.1176/appi.ajp.2007.05122032

Golic, M., Aiff, H., Attman, P. O., Ramsauer, B., Schön, S., Steingrimsson, S., & Svedlund, J. (2023). Lifetime risk of severe kidney disease in lithium-treated patients: A retrospective study. *International Journal of Bipolar Disorders*, *11*, 39. https://doi.org/10.1186/s40345-023-00319-2

Goodwin, G. M., Bowden, C. L., Calabrese, J. R., Grunze, H., Kasper, S., White, R., Greene, P., & Leadbetter, R. (2004). A pooled analysis of 2 placebo-controlled 18-month trials of lamotrigine and lithium maintenance in bipolar I disorder. *Journal of Clinical Psychiatry*, *65*(3), 432-441. https://doi.org/10.4088/jcp.v65n0321

Goodwin, F. K., & Jamison, K. R. (2007). *Manic-depressive illness: Bipolar disorders and recurrent depression* (2nd ed.). Oxford University Press.

Goodwin, G. M., Haddad, P. M., Ferrier, I. N., Aronson, J. K., Barnes, T. R. H., Cipriani, A., Coghill, D. R., Fazel, S., Geddes, J. R., Grunze, H., Holmes, E. A., Howes, O., Hudson, S., Hunt, N., Jones, I., Macmillan, I. C., McAllister-Williams, H., Miklowitz, D. R., Morriss, R., … Young, A. H. (2016). Evidence-based guidelines for treating bipolar disorder: Revised third edition recommendations from the British Association for Psychopharmacology. *Journal of Psychopharmacology*, *30*(6), 495-553. https://doi.org/10.1177/0269881116636545

Grandjean, E. M., & Aubry, J. M. (2009). Lithium: Updated human knowledge using an evidence-based approach. Part II: Clinical pharmacology and therapeutic monitoring. *CNS Drugs*, *23*(4), 331-349. https://doi.org/10.2165/00023210-200923040-00005

Guberman, A. H., Besag, F. M. C., Brodie, M. J., Dooley, J. M., Duchowny, M. S., Pellock, J. M., Richens, A., Stern, R. S., & Trevathan, E. (1999). Lamotrigine-associated rash: Risk and benefit considerations in adults and children. *Epilepsia*, *40*(7), 985-991. https://doi.org/10.1111/j.1528-1157.1999.tb00807.x

Handler, J. (2009). Lithium and antihypertensive medication: A potentially dangerous interaction. *Journal of Clinical Hypertension*, *11*(12), 738-742. https://doi.org/10.1111/j.1751-7176.2009.00181.x

Haussmann, R., Bauer, M., von Bonin, S., Grof, P., & Lewitzka, U. (2015). Treatment of lithium intoxication: Facing the need for evidence. *International Journal of Bipolar Disorders*, *3*, 23. https://doi.org/10.1186/s40345-015-0040-2

Hayes, J. F., Marston, L., Walters, K., Geddes, J. R., King, M., & Osborn, D. P. J. (2016). Lithium vs. valproate vs. olanzapine vs. quetiapine as maintenance monotherapy for bipolar disorder: A population-based UK cohort study using electronic health records. *World Psychiatry*, *15*(1), 53-58. https://doi.org/10.1002/wps.20298

Hedya, S. A., Avula, A., & Swoboda, H. D. (2023). Lithium toxicity. In *StatPearls*. StatPearls Publishing. https://www.ncbi.nlm.nih.gov/books/NBK499992/

Hernández-Díaz, S., Straub, L., Bateman, B. T., Zhu, Y., Mogun, H., Wisner, K. L., Gray, K. J., Lester, B., McDougle, C. J., DiCesare, E., Pennell, P. B., & Huybrechts, K. F. (2024). Risk of autism after prenatal topiramate, valproate, or lamotrigine exposure. *New England Journal of Medicine*, *390*(12), 1069-1079. https://doi.org/10.1056/NEJMoa2309359

Hirsch, L. J., Weintraub, D. B., Buchsbaum, R., Spencer, H. T., Straka, T., Hager, M., & Resor, S. R. (2006). Predictors of lamotrigine-associated rash. *Epilepsia*, *47*(2), 318-322. https://doi.org/10.1111/j.1528-1167.2006.00423.x

Imaz, M. L., Torra, M., Soy, D., García-Esteve, L., & Martin-Santos, R. (2019). Clinical lactation studies of lithium: A systematic review. *Frontiers in Pharmacology*, *10*, 1005. https://doi.org/10.3389/fphar.2019.01005

Jackson, A., Cavanagh, J., & Scott, J. (2003). A systematic review of manic and depressive prodromes. *Journal of Affective Disorders*, *74*(3), 209-217. https://doi.org/10.1016/s0165-0327(02)00266-5

Jamison, K. R., Gerner, R. H., & Goodwin, F. K. (1979). Patient and physician attitudes toward lithium: Relationship to compliance. *Archives of General Psychiatry*, *36*(8), 866-869. https://doi.org/10.1001/archpsyc.1979.01780080040011

Jefferson, J. W. (2010). A clinician's guide to monitoring kidney function in lithium-treated patients. *Journal of Clinical Psychiatry*, *71*(9), 1153-1157. https://doi.org/10.4088/JCP.09com05043

Jentink, J., Dolk, H., Loane, M. A., Morris, J. K., Wellesley, D., Garne, E., de Jong-van den Berg, L., & EUROCAT Antiepileptic Study Working Group. (2010). Intrauterine exposure to carbamazepine and specific congenital malformations: Systematic review and case-control study. *BMJ, 341*, c6581. https://doi.org/10.1136/bmj.c6581

Johnston, A. M., & Eagles, J. M. (1999). Lithium-associated clinical hypothyroidism: Prevalence and risk factors. *British Journal of Psychiatry, 175*, 336-339. https://doi.org/10.1192/bjp.175.4.336

Judd, L. L., Hubbard, B., Janowsky, D. S., Huey, L. Y., & Attewell, P. A. (1977). The effect of lithium carbonate on affect, mood, and personality of normal subjects. *Archives of General Psychiatry, 34*(3), 346-351. https://doi.org/10.1001/archpsyc.1977.01770150104012

Justo, L. P., Soares, B. G., & Calil, H. M. (2007). Family interventions for bipolar disorder. *Cochrane Database of Systematic Reviews, 4*, CD005167. https://doi.org/10.1002/14651858.CD005167.pub2

Juurlink, D. N., Mamdani, M. M., Kopp, A., Rochon, P. A., Shulman, K. I., & Redelmeier, D. A. (2004). Drug-induced lithium toxicity in the elderly: A population-based study. *Journal of the American Geriatrics Society, 52*(5), 794-798. https://doi.org/10.1111/j.1532-5415.2004.52221.x

Keck, P. E., & McElroy, S. L. (2003). Bipolar disorder, obesity, and pharmacotherapy-associated weight gain. *Journal of Clinical Psychiatry, 64*(12), 1426-1435. https://doi.org/10.4088/jcp.v64n1205

Kessing, L. V., Gerds, T. A., Feldt-Rasmussen, B., Andersen, P. K., & Licht, R. W. (2015). Use of lithium and anticonvulsants and the rate of chronic kidney disease: A nationwide population-based study. *JAMA Psychiatry*,

72(12), 1182-1191. https://doi.org/10.1001/jamapsychiatry.2015.1834

Kessing, L. V., Bauer, M., Nolen, W. A., Severus, E., Goodwin, G. M., & Geddes, J. (2018). Effectiveness of maintenance therapy of lithium vs other mood stabilizers in monotherapy and in combinations: A systematic review of evidence from observational studies. *Bipolar Disorders*, *20*(5), 419-431. https://doi.org/10.1111/bdi.12623

Kibirige, D., Luzinda, K., & Ssekitoleko, R. (2013). Spectrum of lithium induced thyroid abnormalities: A current perspective. *Thyroid Research*, *6*, 3. https://doi.org/10.1186/1756-6614-6-3

Kirkham, E., Skinner, J., Anderson, T., Bazire, S., Twigg, M. J., & Desborough, J. A. (2014). One lithium level greater than 1.0 mmol/L causes an acute decline in eGFR: Findings from a retrospective analysis of a monitoring database. *BMJ Open*, *4*(11), e006020. https://doi.org/10.1136/bmjopen-2014-006020

Kirov, G., Tredget, J., John, R., Owen, M. J., & Lazarus, J. H. (2005). A cross-sectional and a prospective study of thyroid disorders in lithium-treated patients. *Journal of Affective Disorders*, *87*(2-3), 313-317. https://doi.org/10.1016/j.jad.2005.03.010

Lam, D., & Wong, G. (1997). Prodromes, coping strategies, insight and social functioning in bipolar affective disorders. *Psychological Medicine*, *27*(5), 1091-1100. https://doi.org/10.1017/s0033291797005540

Lazarus, J. H. (2009). Lithium and thyroid. *Best Practice and Research Clinical Endocrinology and Metabolism*, *23*(6), 723-733. https://doi.org/10.1016/j.beem.2009.06.002

Livingstone, C., & Rampes, H. (2006). Lithium: A review of its metabolic adverse effects. *Journal of Psychopharmacology*, *20*(3), 347-355. https://doi.org/10.1177/0269881105057515

Malhi, G. S., Tanious, M., Das, P., Coulston, C. M., & Berk, M. (2013). Potential mechanisms of action of lithium in bipolar disorder: Current understanding. *CNS Drugs*, *27*(2), 135-153. https://doi.org/10.1007/s40263-013-0039-0

Malhi, G. S., Gessler, D., & Outhred, T. (2017). The use of lithium for the treatment of bipolar disorder: Recommendations from clinical practice guidelines. *Journal of Affective Disorders*, *217*, 266-280. https://doi.org/10.1016/j.jad.2017.03.052

Mansur, R. B., Brietzke, E., & McIntyre, R. S. (2015). Is there a metabolic-mood syndrome? A review of the relationship between obesity and mood disorders. *Neuroscience and Biobehavioral Reviews*, *52*, 89-104. https://doi.org/10.1016/j.neubiorev.2014.12.017

Markowitz, G. S., Radhakrishnan, J., Kambham, N., Valeri, A. M., Hines, W. H., & D'Agati, V. D. (2000). Lithium nephrotoxicity: A progressive combined glomerular and tubulointerstitial nephropathy. *Journal of the American Society of Nephrology*, *11*(8), 1439-1448. https://doi.org/10.1681/ASN.V1181439

McKnight, R. F., Adida, M., Budge, K., Stockton, S., Goodwin, G. M., & Geddes, J. R. (2012). Lithium toxicity profile: A systematic review and meta-analysis. *The Lancet*, *379*(9817), 721-728. https://doi.org/10.1016/S0140-6736(11)61516-X

Meador, K. J., Baker, G. A., Browning, N., Cohen, M. J., Bromley, R. L., Clayton-Smith, J., Kalayjian, L. A., Kanner, A., Liporace, J. D., Pennell, P. B., Privitera, M., & Loring, D. W. (2013). Fetal antiepileptic drug exposure and cognitive outcomes at age 6 years (NEAD study): A prospective observational study. *The Lancet Neurology*, *12*(3), 244-252. https://doi.org/10.1016/S1474-4422(12)70323-X

Medicines and Healthcare products Regulatory Agency. (2018). *Valproate medicines: Contraindicated in women and girls of childbearing potential unless conditions of Pregnancy Prevention Programme are met* (Drug Safety Update). MHRA.

Medicines and Healthcare products Regulatory Agency. (2023). *Valproate: Organisations to prepare for new regulatory measures for oversight of prescribing to new patients and existing female patients* (National Patient Safety Alert). MHRA.

Medicines and Healthcare products Regulatory Agency. (2024a). *Valproate: New safety and educational materials to support regulatory measures in men and women under 55 years of age* (Drug Safety Update, January 2024). MHRA.

Medicines and Healthcare products Regulatory Agency. (2024b). *Valproate use in men: As a precaution, men and their partners should use effective contraception* (Drug Safety Update, September 2024). MHRA.

Medicines and Healthcare products Regulatory Agency. (2025a). *Valproate: Review by two specialists is required for initiating valproate but not for male patients already taking valproate* (Drug Safety Update, Vol. 18, Issue 7, February 2025). MHRA.

Medicines and Healthcare products Regulatory Agency. (2025b). *Valproate: Updated safety and educational materials to support patient discussion on reproductive risks* (Drug Safety Update, Vol. 18, Issue 11, June 2025). MHRA.

Meehan, A. D., Udumyan, R., Kardell, M., Landén, M., Järhult, J., & Wallin, G. (2018). Lithium-associated hypercalcemia:

Pathophysiology, prevalence, management. *World Journal of Surgery*, *42*(2), 415-424. https://doi.org/10.1007/s00268-017-4328-5

Messenheimer, J., Mullens, E. L., Giorgi, L., & Young, F. (1998). Safety review of adult clinical trial experience with lamotrigine. *Drug Safety*, *18*(4), 281-296. https://doi.org/10.2165/00002018-199818040-00004

Meunier, H., Carraz, G., Meunier, Y., Eymard, P., & Aimard, M. (1963). Propriétés pharmacodynamiques de l'acide n-dipropylacétique. *Thérapie*, *18*, 435-438.

Miklowitz, D. J., George, E. L., Richards, J. A., Simoneau, T. L., & Suddath, R. L. (2003). A randomized study of family-focused psychoeducation and pharmacotherapy in the outpatient management of bipolar disorder. *Archives of General Psychiatry*, *60*(9), 904-912. https://doi.org/10.1001/archpsyc.60.9.904

Miklowitz, D. J., & Chung, B. (2016). Family-focused therapy for bipolar disorder: Reflections on 30 years of research. *Family Process*, *55*(3), 483-499. https://doi.org/10.1111/famp.12237

Miura, T., Noma, H., Furukawa, T. A., Mitsuyasu, H., Tanaka, S., Stockton, S., Salanti, G., Motomura, K., Shimano-Katsuki, S., Leucht, S., Cipriani, A., Geddes, J. R., & Kanba, S. (2014). Comparative efficacy and tolerability of pharmacological treatments in the maintenance treatment of bipolar disorder: A systematic review and network meta-analysis. *The Lancet Psychiatry*, *1*(5), 351-359. https://doi.org/10.1016/S2215-0366(14)70314-1

Mockenhaupt, M., Messenheimer, J., Tennis, P., & Schlingmann, J. (2005). Risk of Stevens-Johnson syndrome and toxic epidermal necrolysis in new users of antiepileptics.

Neurology, *64*(7), 1134-1138. https://doi.org/10.1212/01.WNL.0000156354.20227.F0

Morriss, R. K., Faizal, M. A., Jones, A. P., Williamson, P. R., Bolton, C., & McCarthy, J. P. (2007). Interventions for helping people recognise early signs of recurrence in bipolar disorder. *Cochrane Database of Systematic Reviews, 1*, CD004854. https://doi.org/10.1002/14651858.CD004854.pub2

Mullan, K. A., Anderson, A., Illing, P. T., Kwan, P., Purcell, A. W., & Mifsud, N. A. (2019). HLA-associated antiepileptic drug-induced cutaneous adverse reactions. *HLA*, *93*(6), 417-435. https://doi.org/10.1111/tan.13530

Munk-Olsen, T., Liu, X., Viktorin, A., Brown, H. K., Di Florio, A., D'Onofrio, B. M., Gomes, T., Howard, L. M., Khalifeh, H., Krohn, H., Larsson, H., Lichtenstein, P., Taylor, C. L., Van Kamp, I., Wesseloo, R., Meltzer-Brody, S., Vigod, S. N., & Bergink, V. (2018). Maternal and infant outcomes associated with lithium use in pregnancy: An international collaborative meta-analysis of six cohort studies. *The Lancet Psychiatry*, *5*(8), 644-652. https://doi.org/10.1016/S2215-0366(18)30180-9

National Institute for Health and Care Excellence. (2020). *Antenatal and postnatal mental health: Clinical management and service guidance* (Clinical guideline CG192). NICE. https://www.nice.org.uk/guidance/cg192

National Institute for Health and Care Excellence. (2023). *Bipolar disorder: Assessment and management* (Clinical guideline CG185). NICE. https://www.nice.org.uk/guidance/cg185

National Patient Safety Agency. (2009). *Safer lithium therapy* (Patient Safety Alert NPSA/2009/PSA005). NPSA.

Nederlof, M., Heerdink, E. R., Egberts, A. C. G., Wilting, I., Stoker, L. J., Hoekstra, R., & Kupka, R. W. (2018).

Monitoring of patients treated with lithium for bipolar disorder: An international survey. *International Journal of Bipolar Disorders*, *6*, 12. https://doi.org/10.1186/s40345-018-0120-1

Netto, I., & Phutane, V. H. (2012). Reversible lithium neurotoxicity: Review of the literature. *Primary Care Companion for CNS Disorders*, *14*(1), PCC.11r01197. https://doi.org/10.4088/PCC.11r01197

Newport, D. J., Viguera, A. C., Beach, A. J., Ritchie, J. C., Cohen, L. S., & Stowe, Z. N. (2005). Lithium placental passage and obstetrical outcome: Implications for clinical management during late pregnancy. *American Journal of Psychiatry*, *162*(11), 2162-2170. https://doi.org/10.1176/appi.ajp.162.11.2162

Nolen, W. A., Licht, R. W., Young, A. H., Malhi, G. S., Tohen, M., Vieta, E., Kupka, R. W., Zarate, C., Nielsen, R. E., Baldessarini, R. J., & Severus, E. (2019). What is the optimal serum level for lithium in the maintenance treatment of bipolar disorder? A systematic review and recommendations from the ISBD/IGSLI Task Force on treatment with lithium. *Bipolar Disorders*, *21*(5), 394-409. https://doi.org/10.1111/bdi.12805

Nora, J. J., Nora, A. H., & Toews, W. H. (1974). Lithium, Ebstein's anomaly, and other congenital heart defects. *The Lancet*, *304*(7880), 594-595. https://doi.org/10.1016/s0140-6736(74)91918-7

Ott, M., Stegmayr, B., Salander Renberg, E., & Werneke, U. (2016). Lithium intoxication: Incidence, clinical course and renal function, a population-based retrospective cohort study. *Journal of Psychopharmacology*, *30*(10), 1008-1019. https://doi.org/10.1177/0269881116652577

Pacchiarotti, I., Bond, D. J., Baldessarini, R. J., Nolen, W. A., Grunze, H., Licht, R. W., Post, R. M., Berk, M., Goodwin, G. M., Sachs, G. S., Tondo, L., Findling, R. L., Youngstrom, E. A., Tohen, M., Undurraga, J., González-Pinto, A., Goldberg, J. F., Yildiz, A., Altshuler, L. L., … Vieta, E. (2013). The International Society for Bipolar Disorders (ISBD) task force report on antidepressant use in bipolar disorders. *American Journal of Psychiatry*, *170*(11), 1249-1262. https://doi.org/10.1176/appi.ajp.2013.13020185

Pachet, A. K., & Wisniewski, A. M. (2003). The effects of lithium on cognition: An updated review. *Psychopharmacology*, *170*(3), 225-234. https://doi.org/10.1007/s00213-003-1592-x

Parsaik, A. K., Chaudhary, A., Sharma, S., Delgoffe, B. E., Gabor, R., & Singh, B. (2025). Effects of long-term lithium therapy on kidney functioning in mood disorders: A population-based historical cohort study. *Bipolar Disorders*, *27*(1), 28-35. https://doi.org/10.1111/bdi.13501

Paton, C., Adroer, R., & Barnes, T. R. E. (2013). Monitoring lithium therapy: The impact of a quality improvement programme in the UK. *Bipolar Disorders*, *15*(8), 865-875. https://doi.org/10.1111/bdi.12128

Patorno, E., Huybrechts, K. F., Bateman, B. T., Cohen, J. M., Desai, R. J., Mogun, H., Cohen, L. S., & Hernandez-Diaz, S. (2017). Lithium use in pregnancy and the risk of cardiac malformations. *New England Journal of Medicine*, *376*(23), 2245-2254. https://doi.org/10.1056/NEJMoa1612222

Peck, T., Wong, A., & Norman, E. (2010). Anaesthetic implications of psychoactive drugs. *Continuing Education in Anaesthesia Critical Care and Pain*, *10*(6), 177-181. https://doi.org/10.1093/bjaceaccp/mkq033

Perlick, D. A., Rosenheck, R. A., Miklowitz, D. J., Chessick, C., Wolff, N., Kaczynski, R., Ostacher, M., Patel, J., Desai, R., & STEP-BD Family Experience Collaborative Study Group. (2007). Prevalence and correlates of burden among caregivers of patients with bipolar disorder enrolled in the Systematic Treatment Enhancement Program for Bipolar Disorder. *Bipolar Disorders*, *9*(3), 262-273. https://doi.org/10.1111/j.1399-5618.2007.00365.x

Perry, A., Tarrier, N., Morriss, R., McCarthy, E., & Limb, K. (1999). Randomised controlled trial of efficacy of teaching patients with bipolar disorder to identify early symptoms of relapse and obtain treatment. *BMJ*, *318*(7177), 149-153. https://doi.org/10.1136/bmj.318.7177.149

Perucca, E. (2006). Clinically relevant drug interactions with antiepileptic drugs. *British Journal of Clinical Pharmacology*, *61*(3), 246-255. https://doi.org/10.1111/j.1365-2125.2005.02529.x

Post, R. M., Leverich, G. S., Altshuler, L., & Mikalauskas, K. (1992). Lithium-discontinuation-induced refractoriness: Preliminary observations. *American Journal of Psychiatry*, *149*(12), 1727-1729. https://doi.org/10.1176/ajp.149.12.1727

Post, R. M., Altshuler, L. L., Frye, M. A., Suppes, T., Keck, P. E., McElroy, S. L., Leverich, G. S., Luckenbaugh, D. A., Rowe, M., Pizzarello, S., Kupka, R. W., Grunze, H., & Nolen, W. A. (2010). Complexity of pharmacological treatment required for sustained improvement in outpatients with bipolar disorder. *Journal of Clinical Psychiatry*, *71*(9), 1176-1186. https://doi.org/10.4088/JCP.08m04811yel

Post, R. M. (2018). The new news about lithium: An underutilized treatment in the United States. *Neuropsychopharmacology*, *43*(5), 1174-1179. https://doi.org/10.1038/npp.2017.238

Presne, C., Fakhouri, F., Noël, L. H., Stengel, B., Even, C., Kreis, H., Mignon, F., & Grünfeld, J. P. (2003). Lithium-induced nephropathy: Rate of progression and prognostic factors. *Kidney International*, *64*(2), 585-592. https://doi.org/10.1046/j.1523-1755.2003.00096.x

Ragheb, M. (1990). The clinical significance of lithium and nonsteroidal anti-inflammatory drug interactions. *Journal of Clinical Psychopharmacology*, *10*(5), 350-354. https://doi.org/10.1097/00004714-199010000-00009

Reimers, A., & Brodtkorb, E. (2012). Second-generation antiepileptics and pregnancy: A guide for clinicians. *Expert Review of Neurotherapeutics*, *12*(6), 707-717. https://doi.org/10.1586/ern.12.32

Reimers, A., Brodtkorb, E., & Sabers, A. (2015). Interactions between hormonal contraception and antiepileptic drugs: Clinical and mechanistic considerations. *Seizure*, *28*, 66-70. https://doi.org/10.1016/j.seizure.2015.03.006

Reinares, M., Colom, F., Sánchez-Moreno, J., Torrent, C., Martínez-Arán, A., Comes, M., Goikolea, J. M., Benabarre, A., Salamero, M., & Vieta, E. (2008). Impact of caregiver group psychoeducation on the course and outcome of bipolar patients in remission: A randomized controlled trial. *Bipolar Disorders*, *10*(4), 511-519. https://doi.org/10.1111/j.1399-5618.2008.00588.x

Rej, S., Herrmann, N., & Shulman, K. (2012). The effects of lithium on renal function in older adults: A systematic review. *Journal of Geriatric Psychiatry and Neurology*, *25*(1), 51-61. https://doi.org/10.1177/0891988712436690

Rej, S., Elie, D., Mucsi, I., Looper, K. J., & Segal, M. (2015). Chronic kidney disease in lithium-treated older adults: A review of epidemiology, mechanisms, and implications for the treatment of late-life mood disorders. *Drugs and Aging*, *32*(1), 31-42. https://doi.org/10.1007/s40266-014-0234-9

Robert, E., & Guibaud, P. (1982). Maternal valproic acid and congenital neural tube defects. *The Lancet*, *320*(8304), 937. https://doi.org/10.1016/S0140-6736(82)90908-4

Sachs, G. S., Nierenberg, A. A., Calabrese, J. R., Marangell, L. B., Wisniewski, S. R., Gyulai, L., Friedman, E. S., Bowden, C. L., Fossey, M. D., Ostacher, M. J., Ketter, T. A., Patel, J., Hauser, P., Rapport, D., Martinez, J. M., Allen, M. H., Miklowitz, D. J., Otto, M. W., Dennehy, E. B., & Thase, M. E. (2007). Effectiveness of adjunctive antidepressant treatment for bipolar depression. *New England Journal of Medicine*, *356*(17), 1711-1722. https://doi.org/10.1056/NEJMoa064135

Sajatovic, M., Strejilevich, S. A., Gildengers, A. G., Dols, A., Al Jurdi, R. K., Forester, B. P., Kessing, L. V., Beyer, J., Manes, F., Rej, S., Rosa, A. R., Schouws, S. N. T. M., Tsai, S. Y., Young, R. C., & Shulman, K. I. (2015). A report on older-age bipolar disorder from the International Society for Bipolar Disorders Task Force. *Bipolar Disorders*, *17*(7), 689-704. https://doi.org/10.1111/bdi.12331

Schoretsanitis, G., Nikolakopoulou, A., Guinart, D., Correll, C. U., & Kane, J. M. (2022). Prevalence and incidence of chronic kidney disease and its risk factors in lithium-treated patients: A systematic review and meta-analysis. *Bipolar Disorders*, *24*(3), 264-274. https://doi.org/10.1111/bdi.13154

Schou, M. (1979). Artistic productivity and lithium prophylaxis in manic-depressive illness. *British Journal of Psychiatry*, *135*, 97-103. https://doi.org/10.1192/bjp.135.2.97

Schou, M. (2004). *Lithium treatment of mood disorders: A practical guide* (6th ed.). Karger. https://doi.org/10.1159/isbn.978-3-318-01088-4

Scott, J., & Pope, M. (2002). Nonadherence with mood stabilizers: Prevalence and predictors. *Journal of Clinical Psychiatry, 63*(5), 384-390. https://doi.org/10.4088/jcp.v63n0502

Severus, W. E., Kleindienst, N., Seemüller, F., Frangou, S., Möller, H. J., & Greil, W. (2008). What is the optimal serum lithium level in the long-term treatment of bipolar disorder? A review. *Bipolar Disorders, 10*(2), 231-237. https://doi.org/10.1111/j.1399-5618.2007.00475.x

Severus, E., Taylor, M. J., Sauer, C., Pfennig, A., Ritter, P., Bauer, M., & Geddes, J. R. (2014). Lithium for prevention of mood episodes in bipolar disorders: Systematic review and meta-analysis. *International Journal of Bipolar Disorders, 2*, 15. https://doi.org/10.1186/s40345-014-0015-8

Shine, B., McKnight, R. F., Leaver, L., & Geddes, J. R. (2015). Long-term effects of lithium on renal, thyroid, and parathyroid function: A retrospective analysis of laboratory data. *The Lancet, 386*(9992), 461-468. https://doi.org/10.1016/S0140-6736(14)61842-0

Shulman, K. I., Almeida, O. P., Herrmann, N., Schaffer, A., Strejilevich, S. A., Paternoster, C., Amodeo, S., Dols, A., & Sajatovic, M. (2019). Delphi survey of maintenance lithium treatment in older adults with bipolar disorder: An ISBD task force report. *Bipolar Disorders, 21*(2), 117-123. https://doi.org/10.1111/bdi.12714

Sproule, B. (2002). Lithium in bipolar disorder: Can drug concentrations predict therapeutic effect? *Clinical Pharmacokinetics, 41*(9), 639-660. https://doi.org/10.2165/00003088-200241090-00002

Suppes, T., Baldessarini, R. J., Faedda, G. L., & Tohen, M. (1991). Risk of recurrence following discontinuation of lithium treatment in bipolar disorder. *Archives of General Psychiatry*, *48*(12), 1082-1088. https://doi.org/10.1001/archpsyc.1991.01810360046007

Szalat, A., Mazeh, H., & Freund, H. R. (2009). Lithium-associated hyperparathyroidism: Report of four cases and review of the literature. *European Journal of Endocrinology*, *160*(2), 317-323. https://doi.org/10.1530/EJE-08-0620

Timmer, R. T., & Sands, J. M. (1999). Lithium intoxication. *Journal of the American Society of Nephrology*, *10*(3), 666-674. https://doi.org/10.1681/ASN.V103666

Tohen, M., Castillo, J., Baldessarini, R. J., Zarate, C., & Kando, J. C. (1995). Blood dyscrasias with carbamazepine and valproate: A pharmacoepidemiological study of 2,228 patients at risk. *American Journal of Psychiatry*, *152*(3), 413-418. https://doi.org/10.1176/ajp.152.3.413

Tomson, T., Battino, D., Bonizzoni, E., Craig, J., Lindhout, D., Perucca, E., Sabers, A., Thomas, S. V., Vajda, F., & EURAP Study Group. (2018). Comparative risk of major congenital malformations with eight different antiepileptic drugs: A prospective cohort study of the EURAP registry. *The Lancet Neurology*, *17*(6), 530-538. https://doi.org/10.1016/S1474-4422(18)30107-8

Tondo, L., Baldessarini, R. J., Hennen, J., Floris, G., Silvetti, F., & Tohen, M. (1998). Lithium treatment and risk of suicidal behavior in bipolar disorder patients. *Journal of Clinical Psychiatry*, *59*(8), 405-414. https://doi.org/10.4088/jcp.v59n0802

Tondo, L., Abramowicz, M., Alda, M., Bauer, M., Bocchetta, A., Bolzani, L., Calkin, C. V., Chillotti, C., Hidalgo-Mazzei, D., Manchia, M., Müller-Oerlinghausen, B., Murru, A., Perugi,

G., Pinna, M., Quaranta, G., Reginaldi, D., Reif, A., Ritter, P., Rybakowski, J. K., … Baldessarini, R. J. (2017). Long-term lithium treatment in bipolar disorder: Effects on glomerular filtration rate and other metabolic parameters. *International Journal of Bipolar Disorders*, *5*, 27. https://doi.org/10.1186/s40345-017-0096-2

Torrent, C., Amann, B., Sánchez-Moreno, J., Colom, F., Reinares, M., Comes, M., Rosa, A. R., & Vieta, E. (2008). Weight gain in bipolar disorder: Pharmacological treatment as a contributing factor. *Acta Psychiatrica Scandinavica*, *118*(1), 4-18. https://doi.org/10.1111/j.1600-0447.2008.01204.x

Van Amelsvoort, T., Bakshi, R., Devaux, C. B., & Schwabe, S. (1994). Hyponatremia associated with carbamazepine and oxcarbazepine therapy: A review. *Epilepsia*, *35*(1), 181-188. https://doi.org/10.1111/j.1528-1157.1994.tb02930.x

Vendsborg, P. B., Bech, P., & Rafaelsen, O. J. (1976). Lithium treatment and weight gain. *Acta Psychiatrica Scandinavica*, *53*(2), 139-147. https://doi.org/10.1111/j.1600-0447.1976.tb00068.x

Viguera, A. C., Whitfield, T., Baldessarini, R. J., Newport, D. J., Stowe, Z., Reminick, A., Zurick, A., & Cohen, L. S. (2007). Risk of recurrence in women with bipolar disorder during pregnancy: Prospective study of mood stabilizer discontinuation. *American Journal of Psychiatry*, *164*(12), 1817-1824. https://doi.org/10.1176/appi.ajp.2007.06101639

Viguera, A. C., Whitfield, T., Baldessarini, R. J., Newport, D. J., Stowe, Z., Reminick, A., Zurick, A., & Cohen, L. S. (2007a). Risk of recurrence in women with bipolar disorder during pregnancy: Prospective study of mood stabilizer discontinuation. *American Journal of Psychiatry*, *164*(12), 1817-1824. https://doi.org/10.1176/appi.ajp.2007.06101639

Viguera, A. C., Newport, D. J., Ritchie, J., Stowe, Z., Whitfield, T., Mogielnicki, J., Baldessarini, R. J., Zurick, A., & Cohen, L. S. (2007b). Lithium in breast milk and nursing infants: Clinical implications. *American Journal of Psychiatry, 164*(2), 342-345. https://doi.org/10.1176/ajp.2007.164.2.342

Viktorin, A., Lichtenstein, P., Thase, M. E., Larsson, H., Lundholm, C., Magnusson, P. K. E., & Landén, M. (2014). The risk of switch to mania in patients with bipolar disorder during treatment with an antidepressant alone and in combination with a mood stabilizer. *American Journal of Psychiatry, 171*(10), 1067-1073. https://doi.org/10.1176/appi.ajp.2014.13111501

Wang, X. Q., Lang, S. Y., Shi, X. B., Tian, H. J., Wang, R. F., & Yang, F. (2010). Cross-reactivity of skin rashes with current antiepileptic drugs in Chinese population. *Seizure, 19*(9), 562-566. https://doi.org/10.1016/j.seizure.2010.09.003

Waring, W. S. (2006). Management of lithium toxicity. *Toxicological Reviews, 25*(4), 221-230. https://doi.org/10.2165/00139709-200625040-00003

Weintraub, D., Buchsbaum, R., Resor, S. R., & Hirsch, L. J. (2007). Psychiatric and behavioral side effects of the newer antiepileptic drugs in adults with epilepsy. *Epilepsy & Behavior, 10*(1), 105-110. https://doi.org/10.1016/j.yebeh.2006.08.008

Weisler, R. H., Kalali, A. H., Ketter, T. A., & SPD417 Study Group. (2004). A multicenter, randomized, double-blind, placebo-controlled trial of extended-release carbamazepine capsules as monotherapy for bipolar disorder patients with manic or mixed episodes. *Journal of Clinical Psychiatry, 65*(4), 478-484. https://doi.org/10.4088/jcp.v65n0405

Werneke, U., Ott, M., Renberg, E. S., Taylor, D., & Stegmayr, B. (2012). A decision analysis of long-term lithium treatment and the risk of renal failure. *Acta Psychiatrica Scandinavica*, *126*(3), 186-197. https://doi.org/10.1111/j.1600-0447.2012.01847.x

Wesseloo, R., Kamperman, A. M., Munk-Olsen, T., Pop, V. J. M., Kushner, S. A., & Bergink, V. (2016). Risk of postpartum relapse in bipolar disorder and postpartum psychosis: A systematic review and meta-analysis. *American Journal of Psychiatry*, *173*(2), 117-127. https://doi.org/10.1176/appi.ajp.2015.15010124

Wesseloo, R., Wierdsma, A. I., van Kamp, I. L., Munk-Olsen, T., Hoogendijk, W. J. G., Kushner, S. A., & Bergink, V. (2017). Lithium dosing strategies during pregnancy and the postpartum period. *British Journal of Psychiatry*, *211*(1), 31-36. https://doi.org/10.1192/bjp.bp.116.192799

Weston, J., Bromley, R., Jackson, C. F., Adab, N., Clayton-Smith, J., Greenhalgh, J., Hounsome, J., McKay, A. J., Tudur Smith, C., & Marson, A. G. (2016). Monotherapy treatment of epilepsy in pregnancy: Congenital malformation outcomes in the child. *Cochrane Database of Systematic Reviews*, *11*, CD010224. https://doi.org/10.1002/14651858.CD010224.pub2

Wieck, A., & Jones, S. (2018). Dangers of valproate in pregnancy. *BMJ*, *361*, k1609. https://doi.org/10.1136/bmj.k1609

Wingo, A. P., Wingo, T. S., Harvey, P. D., & Baranyi, J. (2009). Effects of lithium on cognitive performance: A meta-analysis. *Journal of Clinical Psychiatry*, *70*(11), 1588-1597. https://doi.org/10.4088/JCP.08r04972

Yatham, L. N., Kennedy, S. H., Parikh, S. V., Schaffer, A., Bond, D. J., Frey, B. N., Sharma, V., Goldstein, B. I., Rej, S., Beaulieu, S., Alda, M., MacQueen, G., Milev, R. V.,

Ravindran, A., O'Donovan, C., McIntosh, D., Lam, R. W., Vazquez, G., Kapczinski, F., … Berk, M. (2018). Canadian Network for Mood and Anxiety Treatments (CANMAT) and International Society for Bipolar Disorders (ISBD) 2018 guidelines for the management of patients with bipolar disorder. *Bipolar Disorders*, *20*(2), 97-170. https://doi.org/10.1111/bdi.12609

About the Author

Timothy Sawyer Duncan writes about medicine for the people it happens to.

His books deal with the distance between what the research shows and what patients are actually told. That distance is where most of the damage occurs: treatments with thin evidence and loud advocates, conditions that get dismissed rather than investigated, and appointments in which a well-informed person still cannot get a hearing. He works from the primary literature rather than from summaries of it, and he reports the studies that came back negative alongside the ones that did not, on the view that a reader handed only a promise has been sold something rather than informed.

He accepts no funding, sponsorship, speaking fees, or commissions from pharmaceutical manufacturers, compounding pharmacies, telehealth services, treatment providers, or patient advocacy organizations, and holds no financial interest in any treatment described in his books.

He writes for the reader who would rather have an accurate picture than a comfortable one.

www.ingramcontent.com/pod-product-compliance
Lightning Source LLC
LaVergne TN
LVHW052325200926
848481LV00002B/676
* 9 7 9 8 9 0 5 9 9 3 0 3 9 *